THE PATH OF THE YOGA SUTRAS

Also by Nicolai Bachman

The Language of Yoga

The Yoga Sutras (a home-study course)

The Path of the Yoga Sutras

a practical guide to the core of yoga

NICOLAI BACHMAN

Sounds True
BOULDER, COLORADO

Sounds True, Inc.,
Boulder, Colorado 80306

Published 2011

Cover and book design by Rachael Murray
Cover art © Andrea Haase from shutterstock.com
Author photo (page 271) © Jennifer Esperanza

FSC
www.fsc.org
MIX
Paper from responsible sources
FSC® C016245

The wood used to produce this book is from Forest Stewardship Council (FSC) certified forests, recycled materials, or controlled wood.

Printed in Canada

Library of Congress Cataloging-in-Publication Data
Bachman, Nicolai.
The path of the yoga sutras : a practical guide to the core of yoga / by Nicolai Bachman.
p. cm.
Includes bibliographical references and index.
ISBN 978-1-60407-429-1
1. Yoga. I. Title.
B132.Y6B26 2011
181'.45--dc22

2011007104

eBook ISBN 978-1-60407-472-7

15

To all teachers who have shared their wisdom and experience, who have walked their talk, and who have quietly opened our hearts and minds to the pure inner spirit residing within each of us. *Praṇāma!* (Respectful blessings to you!)

Out beyond ideas of wrongdoing and rightdoing,
there is a field. I'll meet you there.

RUMI, from SOUL, HEART, AND BODY ONE MORNING

CONTENTS

Foreword by Tias Little xiii
Preface xix
Acknowledgments xxi

Introduction 1

PART 1: KEY PRINCIPLES

1 Atha *Readiness and Commitment* 7
2 Citta *Heart-Mind Field of Consciousness* 11
3 Puruṣa *Pure Inner Light of Awareness* 17
4 Dṛśya *Ever-Changing Mother Nature* 21
5 Viveka *Keen Discernment* 25
6 Abhyāsa *Diligent, Focused Practice* 29
7 Vairāgya *Nonattachment to Sensory Objects* 33
8 Yoga as Nirodha *Silencing the Heart-Mind* 39
9 Īśvara *The Source of Knowledge* 43
10 Karma and Saṁskāra *Action and Its Imprint* 49
11 Pariṇāma *Transformation* 57

PART 2: UNDERSTANDING SUFFERING

12 Duḥkha *Suffering as Opportunity* 65
13 Saṁyoga *False Identification of the Seer with the Seen* 71
14 Vṛtti-s *Activity in the Heart-Mind* 75
15 Pramāṇa *Correct Evaluation* 79
16 Viparyaya *Misperception* 83
17 Vikalpa *Imagination* 87
18 Nidrā *Sleep* 91
19 Smṛti *Memory* 95
20 Antarāya-s *Obstacles That Distract* 99
21 Kleśa-s *Mental-Emotional Afflictions* 105
22 Avidyā *Lack of Awareness* 109
23 Asmitā *Distorted Sense of Self* 113
24 Rāga *Clinging to Past Pleasure* 119
25 Dveṣa *Clinging to Past Suffering* 123
26 Abhiniveśa *Fear of Death* 129

PART 3: OUTER BEHAVIOR

27 Aṣṭāṅga *The Eight Limbs of Yoga* 135
28 Yama-s *Ethical Practices* 139
29 Ahiṁsā *Nonviolence and Compassion* 143
30 Satya *Truthfulness and Sincerity* 149
31 Asteya *Not Taking from Others* 153
32 Brahmacarya *Conservation of Vital Energy* 157
33 Aparigraha *Nonhoarding* 161
34 Pratipakṣa-Bhāvana *Cultivating the Opposite* 165

PART 4: PERSONAL PRACTICES

35 Niyama-s *Personal Self-Care* 171
36 Śauca *Cleanliness* 175
37 Santoṣa *Contentment and Gratitude* 179
38 Kriyā-Yoga *Practice in Action* 185
39 Tapas *Practice Causing Positive Change* 189
40 Svādhyāya *Study by and of Oneself* 195
41 Īśvara-Praṇidhāna *Humility and Faith* 201
42 Āsana *Refinement of the Body* 207
43 Prāṇāyāma *Regulation of Breath* 211

PART 5: INNER DEVELOPMENT

44 Pratyāhāra *Tuning Out Sensory Input* 217
45 Citta-Prasādana *Purification of the Heart-Mind* 221
46 Dhāraṇā *Choosing a Focus* 227
47 Dhyāna *Continuous Focus* 231
48 Samādhi *Complete Attention* 235
49 Saṁyama *Focusing Inward* 241
50 Pratiprasava *Returning to the Source* 245
51 Kaivalya *Permanent Oneness* 249

Epilogue 253
Permissions and Credits 255
For Further Study 257
Further Resources 259
Index 261
About the Author 271

FOREWORD

AT THE OUTSET OF MY training as an early twenty-something, I was eager, enthusiastic, and passionate for the discipline of yoga. After a trip to India in 1989, my curiosity accelerated, yet I was uncertain about how to connect to the greater yoga tradition in a more in-depth and sustained way. It was not until I was introduced to the Sanskrit language with Nicolai Bachman that I found a foothold in the long, and at times sheer, climb up the yoga mountain. Blessed to find Nicolai as a teacher, I came to see how the yoga experience is intimately connected to sound and vibration. Not only is Sanskrit the source of the vast and subtle knowledge pertaining to yoga, but it relates to the direct experience within yoga, whether through memorization of a *sūtra*, the intonation of mantra, or the vibration that pulses through the body's energy channels (*nāḍī-s*) in yoga postures. As I continue to study with Nicolai today, it is not just the mechanics of Sanskrit that he elucidates, but the mystical and energetic associations pertaining to the language.

The Yoga Sūtras of Patañjali are built on the Sanskrit language, and in many respects they are the bedrock for yoga training. In this book, Nicolai does a great service of unpacking the weight of the Sanskrit so that traveling the terrain of the Yoga Sūtras is clear and easy to follow.

Over the years, Nicolai and I have deciphered the *sūtra-s* together on long treks in the mountains of northern New

Mexico—he parsing out the vocabulary and meaning, while I contributed my experience on the mat and on the meditation cushion. Given that the yogic journey is in many respects a solitary one, it has been a unique and invaluable opportunity for me to share an investigation into the yoga teachings with my colleague and friend Nicolai.

Inspired by Nicolai—and through my own investigations into the roots of the yoga teachings—it has become clear to me that a dedicated yoga practice must not be limited to the execution of physical postures and should involve a close investigation of activity within the mind-heart. It is ironic that, today, yoga has become identified with flexible hamstrings and abdominal lifts, for historically it has involved careful and extensive analysis of thought, feeling, attitude, and point of view.

At the heart of yoga practice is inquiry. In order for human beings to transform in positive ways involving mind, body, and emotion, there must be some critical means of self-reflection. In the following chapters, Nicolai unravels the *sūtra-s*, not only from his vantage point of the Sanskrit language, but from the depths of his own study, inquiry, and practice.

The Yoga Sūtras of Patañjali is a gateway into the realm of inquiry, and for the committed yoga student it offers a vocabulary to begin to see into patterns of emotional and psychological holding. The *sūtra-s* are threads— and sometimes but strands of thread—that require a guide or coach to help unravel them due to the terse, minimalist style in which they are rendered. In the pages ahead, Nicolai takes some of the complex and difficult-to-grasp themes within the *sūtra-s* and renders them more accessible. The *sūtra-s* are not intentionally cryptic or out of reach in the way that *koans* are in the Chinese and Japanese traditions. In keeping with the greater *sūtra* tradition, Patañjali's Yoga Sūtras invite commentary. Like a Rubik's Cube, the *sūtra-s* are meant to be turned over, examined, tested, and aligned until the practitioner realizes the complete mandala of the Cube.

So inquiry or investigative self-reflection is the basis for yogic maturation and ultimately the means to self-knowledge. If a yoga practice is devoid of inquiry into the nature of mind or devoid of real self-reflection, is it really yoga?

In guiding us through the *sūtra-s*, Nicolai takes the overall grid of the *sūtra-s* and elucidates the most integral and elemental patterns within the text. This is extremely helpful, for the Yoga Sūtras of Patañjali are wide in scope and include an array of different means to the direct experience of yoga. The teaching within each *sūtra* connects to the "field" of the other *sūtra-s*. It is this way in the body as well. That is, the shoulder blade is connected to the sacrum via connective tissue, and the tongue has ligamentous and energetic connections to the respiratory diaphragm. I like to think of the *sūtra-s* as a "field," like an electromagnetic field, and each verse connects to the verse that precedes and follows it, and also to other verses within the field. This is why the thematic groupings of the concepts offered in the following chapters, such as *karma*, suffering, practice, restraint, and meditation give us clues about how to find our way into the mandala of the *sūtra-s* and to understand their essential patterns.

It is possible to approach Patañjali's *sūtra-s* as a philosophical puzzle that must be interpreted and understood intellectually. And while the text is heuristic (in keeping with the rich and vibrant yoga tradition that involved extensive debate, reasoning, and logic), it is also meant to be a practical guide for personal transformation. Rather than exercises in mental abstraction however, the *sūtra-s*, if they are to be effective stratagems for change, must be actualized and lived. It is in this spirit that this book renders the verses of the Yoga Sūtras. Nicolai breathes life into the teachings, and through a candid, clear-eyed approach, he makes the principles within the text applicable and workable in everyday life.

On our long walks in the Sangre de Cristo Mountains outside of Santa Fe, Nicolai and I have explored the heart of the yoga teachings. In the way that a turn on the trail offers a new vista, our dialogues attempt to view the teachings from as many points of view as possible. Trekking on a path, be it a mountain path or a spiritual path, is made possible by those travelers who precede us. Once the path is cleared of tangled overgrowth and debris, it is easier to make progress. The *sūtra-s* of Patañjali do just this. By elucidating the hazards of emotional and psychological clinging, they allow for passage on the path of yoga, thus clearing the way toward spiritual fulfillment. The journey is profoundly an inward one. Patañjali guides one on a pilgrimage through the jungles of distraction and confusion in the heart-mind to the inner sanctum of the seer or witness.

As a friend and colleague, I know Nicolai's greatest asset to be his capacity to discriminate—clearly, objectively, and lovingly. This capacity for discernment is central to the teachings of Patañjali. In the Yoga Sūtras, the instrument to freeing the mind, body, and spirit is discriminating awareness. The sword of discrimination is used to disentangle the pure witness from the everyday perceiver with its mixed bag of perceptions, mental chatter, dreams, and habitual psychological tendencies.

To make progress on the path, the yogi must have the sword of discrimination held up high, with a readiness to cut through. The Yoga Sūtras inspire practitioners to keep their blade of discriminatory awareness sharp. The edge inevitably grows dull. Today there is greater opportunity for self-indulgence and interconnectedness alike, given the onslaught of the digital age and the influence of the media where youth and adults alike whittle away their time on cellular devices and broadband networks. Those dedicated to the path of yoga through practice and engaged insight must daily sharpen their blade. The yogi and yogini hone the sword of good judgment via the whetstone of the breath, the precision and flow of the yoga posture, the subtle adjustments of the diaphragm and respiratory muscles in *prāṇāyāma*, and careful insight (*vipassana*) into the moods, thoughts, and opinions that surface in meditation. This acumen cuts away the ingrown thoughts that cause affliction and deteriorate the force of *prāṇa* inside; it also gives balance and integrity to one's relationships in the world. When intentions are infused with attitudes of nonharming and kindness, when the yogi is conciliate in dialogue and personal action, then there is a greater possibility for personal and societal peace. These intentions are at the foot of the eight-limbed path within Patañjali's yoga (*yama* and *niyama*), and by realizing them the yogi is closer to the trail's end of enlightened awareness.

The metaphor of the sword is utilized throughout the spiritual disciplines of Asia. It is suggestive of battle and the pose of the warrior. However, the yogi is not inclined to unsheathe his or her sword in order to brandish it upon others but utilizes the sword inwardly to excise bias, selfishness, and myopic thinking. This sword of discrimination is to be used mindfully and with great care. A buddhist teacher once wrote, "My only weapon is the weapon of gentleness." May all beings embody this potent combination: sharp sword, open heart.

When teaching yoga postures, I frequently describe the body using the analogy of a cairn—a tier of rocks piled vertically to reveal the presence of a hiking trail or to mark the location of something significant. I liken the pelvis, spine, and cranium to that tier of stones. When the first several stones at the base—the pelvis and lumbar spine—are in place, there can be stability and lightness above.

In *The Path of the Yoga Sūtras*, Nicolai guides us through the *sūtra-s* by delineating the path via a series of helpful cairns. Given the wilderness of Sanskrit terminology and minimalist rendering of its yoga philosophy, it is easy to lose one's way. Nicolai charts a course through the *sūtra-s* that is invaluable for the reader. The descriptions of the *sūtra-s* in this collection are clearly marked. In the way that a cairn is a heartwarming sight on the trail as dusk approaches and shadows are looming, the pointers in this guide inspire confidence and trust. May this book be a resource for all students of yoga to progress on their path with greater fortitude, certainty, and joy.

Tias Little
Prajna Yoga
Santa Fe, New Mexico
April 2011

PREFACE

IF YOU ARE INTERESTED IN learning about the core of who you are, and how that core affects your everyday relationships, perceptions, and actions, then the principles and practices described in the Yoga Sūtras can help. The text provides a theoretical structure of human consciousness, with directions on how to navigate our way through life's ups and downs. Emphasis is laid on turning our attention inward to more fully understand what our true nature is all about. Who are we now? How can we become more happy and fulfilled human beings?

I came to study the Yoga Sūtras from a background in yoga *āsana*, meditation, and Sanskrit. After reading several different translations and still not feeling comfortable with my understanding, I sought out qualified teachers who had themselves studied the Yoga Sūtras over many years with their teachers, and had applied the principles and practices to their lives. For me, this was the key that unlocked the door. There is no substitute for having a kind, knowledgeable, inspiring teacher who walks the talk.

Integrating yoga philosophy into my life was also absolutely necessary. Yoga is meant to be experiential, not just intellectual. Yet it was asking questions of my primary teachers that caused the proverbial light bulbs to brighten my understanding.

I personally appreciate the Yoga Sūtras as much for its masterful design as for its universality and emphasis on personal growth. The ideas espoused in the text, such as truthfulness, self-observation, and diligent practice, are truly independent of time, place, culture, or religion. The author, Patañjali, offers unique and powerful tools for inner development and outer poise. These include living a kind, civil life; refining the body, mind, and sense organs; and turning our attention inward to understand the true nature of the inner Self.

Learning the concepts and implementing the practices of yoga is a lifelong pursuit that is bound to create outer joy and inner happiness. The ability to catch myself before I act unconsciously, based on past habitual patterning, then deciding to change course and act in a beneficial and positive way, makes me appreciate the usefulness and profundity of the Yoga Sūtras. Every time I am able to listen to all sides of an argument or see another person as a manifestation of the radiant light of awareness that we all share, I am reminded of how powerful and transformative the practices are. These are just a few of many, many examples where this wisdom can be applied.

Remember, the purpose of yoga is clarification of our individual field of consciousness in order to perceive external events clearly and connect to our inner light of awareness, our inner Self. Spiritual development involves conscious change and refinement—replacing one's unconscious, negative habitual patterns with conscious, positive, helpful practices that dissolve attachments and lead to a healthier, happier being.

ACKNOWLEDGMENTS

ALL OF US ENCOUNTER CERTAIN people in our lives who deeply influence who we are, how we think and what we do. For me, first and foremost are my parents. My mother, Brigitte—always interested in what is best for her children—continues to provide steadfast love, nurturance, and wise counsel. My father, Charles—a poet and philosopher by nature—is able to slow down, listen, and give his full attention to whomever he spends time with. He has always encouraged me to follow my heart. My wife, Margo, whose constant love and support of our whole family allowed me to carve out the time and space to write. Her clear and compassionate communication has been extraordinary. Margo, I love you and cherish our partnership. My children, Sierra and Mateo, are my teachers from whom I learn every day. My brother and close friend Eric is a shining example of how brains, brawn, and kindness are possible in a single human being.

Friends and teachers who have been a blessing in my life include Denise Larosa, Sonam Willow, Dr. Vasant Lad, Claudia Welch, Will Foster, Vyaas Houston, Vagish Shastri, David Frawley, and Sonia Nelson. I am so very grateful for the utterly enjoyable, stimulating, and illuminating company of my close friend and colleague Tias Little, who has supported my work for so many years. Our conversations in the mountains and high-desert trails around Santa Fe continue to fuel new ideas and possibilities.

Thank you to all of my friends and students who continue to teach me every time we interact, and to the staff of Sounds True for believing in what I have to offer.

Finally, for proofreading the text, I would like to thank my wife, Margo; Pat Shapiro; my father, Charles Bachman; and Tias Little.

INTRODUCTION

PATAÑJALI, THE AUTHOR OF the Yoga Sūtras, lived somewhere between 500 BCE and 200 CE, a time that possibly overlaps the life of Buddha and a period of intense philosophical activity in India. Patañjali was revered as an outstanding scholar and wise man who wrote significant commentaries on Sanskrit grammar and Āyurveda (East Indian medicine). So much was he praised that he became deified as a sort of prophet, an incarnation of God in the form of Viṣṇu and also Ādiśeṣa, the thousand-headed serpent whose coils provide a bed for Viṣṇu to rest on.

Yoga itself existed long before Patañjali. He did not create yoga, but he brilliantly compiled its essence in a text called *Pātañjala-Yoga-Darśanam*, meaning "view of yoga according to Patañjali." The Patañjali yoga tradition is a later expression of older teachings based on the source texts of India known as the Veda-s, which date earlier than 1500 BCE. Yoga is considered one of the six "views," or perspectives, on the same basic Vedic philosophy.

The Yoga Sūtras came to be accepted as the primary text on yoga philosophy, not yoga postures (*āsana*). Patañjali focuses on yoga as a method of transforming the way we think, communicate, and act by directing our attention inward and cultivating inner contentment. Less than 2 percent of the *sūtra-s* discuss the physical practice of *āsana*. In fact, according to what those few *sūtra-s* say, we could interpret *āsana* as simply how to sit for meditation. So yoga is much, much more than *āsana*.

The Yoga Sūtras consists of 195 small, concise aphorisms (called *sūtra-s*) in four chapters. The aphorisms are written in Sanskrit, a language designed to express the subtle aspects of yoga. The text describes human consciousness in detail, including how our heart-mind functions, how suffering happens, and how to refine our body, breath, mind, and heart so we are able to cultivate inner happiness and free ourselves from negativity.

There has been an unbroken oral transmission of information in India for thousands of years. To facilitate the memorization of information, the *sūtra* "thread" format was invented, in which a large amount of knowledge is expressed in a short phrase or sentence. Many of these aphorisms strung together create a text on the topic at hand. Thus, one can establish a mnemonic association between the tiny, memorized *sūtra* and all of the knowledge associated with it that was received from a teacher. Traditionally the sound of a text is learned by heart first, through chanting, then the meaning is taught and applied to a well-rounded practice of all eight limbs of yoga.

Usually, there was one teacher with a small class of young students learning together. The teacher would test students occasionally to see if they were doing their practice and applying the principles outside of class. It was the students' responsibility to apply the ideas and practices outside of class. For example, let's say a posture is taught one day. The students are expected to practice that posture regularly. If students return with questions about it, or they have noticeably improved their form, it is obvious to the teacher that they have spent some time with it. On the other hand, if other students are making no observable progress, they will fall behind. Studious and hard-working students will move forward and receive deeper instruction, while those who are apathetic or lazy will eventually drop out. No teacher wants to waste their time with inattentive students.

Traditionally, students may live with a teacher for many years, studying all day, every day, in order to master a subject, be it philosophy, music, dance, or other discipline. In ancient India and even today, there are teachers who are supported by the greater community and do not expect payment from students. Respect for the teacher is required, and honoring a power higher than ourselves (usually in the form of a deity) is a powerful way to prevent the ego from taking over.

Eventually, the students will become teachers or performers, and if fame follows, it is absolutely essential that humility is ingrained in their consciousness. Many teachers want nothing more than for one of their students to surpass them and, thus, carry on their teachings. Master teachers have the knowledge fully integrated into their being.

Integrating the teachings of yoga means experiencing them outside and inside ourselves. Civil and kind social interaction; caring for, developing, and stabilizing our physical body and breath; self-observation; quiet contemplation; and deep meditation all contribute to the clarification of our heart-mind. As our sensory organs become clear and acute, we perceive objects as they truly are. When we are able to focus our attention away from the external and toward our inner core, then we can connect to that pure inner light of awareness that all creatures share. Yoga is the process of stilling (*nirodha*) the distractions in our heart-mind.

The Sanskrit word *sattva* is very important to understand in the context of yoga. *Sattva* represents what is universally accepted as good and positive. Its qualities include love, compassion, wisdom, intelligence, truthfulness, radiance, purity, harmony, balance, nonviolence, virtue, appropriateness, and adaptability. Being *sattvic* means acting according to *sattva*, knowing when and how to act for the greater good, and not being attached to the results of our actions. As our heart-mind becomes more refined through the practices and processes of yoga, it gradually becomes more and more *sattvic.*

THIS APPROACH TO LEARNING YOGA

The almost two hundred *sūtra-s* can be difficult to grasp when approached linearly, one after another. Here, I have carefully selected fifty-one key principles of yoga to focus on and explore in depth. Rather than gleaning pieces of each principle by moving through the text in a linear way, we can instead see all aspects of it in one place. All of the significant principles of yoga are encased in Sanskrit words, most of which have no English equivalent. Learning what yoga is all about requires understanding these core principles intellectually and experientially. Each principle is explained in its own chapter that includes real-life examples, thoughts to meditate on, and exercises to apply it into your life. Acquiring this basic vocabulary of yoga will enable you to converse with others using the Sanskrit words instead of awkward English approximations. Discussing these ideas with others will greatly broaden your understanding of them. Patience is key. The principles and practices of yoga will seep into your system as you study and integrate them over time.

The concepts are ordered to build on each other. Focusing on one chapter at a time will allow your heart and mind time to integrate each concept fully. Contemplate each thought deeply and quietly, and practice the exercises to experience what the concept means to you. Spend time on each concept, as you would a long, drawn-out meal, and you will be able to fully digest it. Choose the exercises that will benefit you the most. Learning the principles of yoga will expand and deepen your *āsana* practice.

PART 1

KEY PRINCIPLES

1

ATHA

Readiness and Commitment

अथ

Until one is committed, there is a hesitancy, the chance
to draw back. The moment one definitely commits oneself
then Providence moves too. All sorts of things occur to
help one that would otherwise never have occurred.
Whatever you can do, or dream you can, *begin it.*
Boldness has genius, power and magic in it.

JOHANN WOLFGANG VON GOETHE

BEGINNINGS, LIKE ENDINGS, CAN BE difficult or exciting. Starting something new implies change, a step toward an eventual goal. *Atha* is the very first word in the Yoga Sūtras and is considered an auspicious way to begin. Whenever we make an important decision, often the universe will energetically support us.

Atha here means beginning the study of who we are, where we are, and how we can make incremental changes to our inner and outer self in order to be less involved with material objects and more in tune with how we feel and how our actions affect those around us.

Learning, practicing, and integrating the various aspects of yoga happens over a long period of time and requires patience and perseverance. Beware: your initial eagerness and energy may not last. Allow the information to seep into your core gradually and intentionally. There is no rush. Many of us want instant gratification—to learn something and then quickly move on to something else. Yet real, lasting inner change takes time.

Our eagerness to learn and the frequency of our practice will affect the velocity of learning. A person can be extremely excited to learn yoga, yet not have the discipline to follow through with the practices. If we are enrolled in a class because it is required for our degree or certificate, we may fall into boredom or become lackadaisical. Practicing often but in an inattentive way will also hamper progress. Ideally, we genuinely want to learn, are able to carve out time in our schedule to learn, and can maintain a regular and consistent practice for long enough to allow the knowledge we seek to sink in.

A heart-mind that is fresh and open will absorb information like a sponge. Repetition reinforces the knowledge learned by creating a pattern in the heart-mind. Young children are a perfect example of open heart-minds learning through repetition. Not only do they have less in their hearts and minds to interfere with perception, but they will also repeat something over and over to themselves until it sticks (leaves a lasting impression) in their memory. Growing up, we accumulate obstacles to learning in the form of physical limitations, emotional scars, and intellectual or spiritual rigidity. Cultivating a beginner's mind during our studies will allow us to truly grasp the profound depths of yoga.

The Internet avails us to almost unlimited amounts of information. With so many different directions to choose from, how can we focus on those that improve our lives? Sitting in a restful state of quietness allows us to observe the crazy movements of the world. Regrouping, then setting an intention and deciding to follow one particular direction, will open up opportunities that otherwise would not have been available. Similarly, prayer lets the universe know how to help us.

Sometimes we bite off more than we can chew by taking on too many projects. This can create more stress for us and siphons our attention from our friends and family. It is important to sit quietly and contemplate whether we have the time and resources to commit to another endeavor. For example, a decision to have children requires that you let go of certain activities in order to give your children the attention they need to grow up healthy and happy. All of a sudden, your priorities have shifted, and a new kind of lifestyle has begun.

Commitment holds a solid, grounding energy that provides stability and structure to our lives. Deciding to learn and experience what yoga really is requires diligence and effort, which will undoubtedly yield fruit over time. Yoga is a lifestyle designed to develop and refine our body, mind, and heart, our thoughts, words, and actions. As Steve Jobs once said, "The journey is the reward."

THOUGHTS

Learning anything well requires eagerness,
commitment, and perseverance.

With an open mind, I can direct my attention
inward and see what unfolds.

I will set aside time for learning and
practicing the principles of yoga.

Exercises

Think of a time when you took on too many projects at the same time. Writing down your thoughts, ask yourself:

Which projects could have waited?

How did this overextended state affect the quality of your personal life?

What could you have done differently?

Think of other areas of study you began, but could not keep up. Write down the reason(s) why you think they ended. Did something more appealing replace them? Did you give them enough of a chance?

What commitments have you made in your life that have brought you fulfillment?

2

CITTA

Heart-Mind Field of Consciousness

चित्त

The Power of the Universe will come to your assistance,
if your heart and mind are in Unity.
LAKOTA SAYING, passed down from WHITE BUFFALO CALF WOMAN

WE ARE ALL CONDITIONED BY our experience. Whenever we see, hear, taste, smell, touch, feel, think, speak, or act, our heart and mind are affected. It is our heart-mind field that accepts sensory input from outside, processes it, integrates it into ourselves, and remembers, ruminates, and directs the delivery of thoughts, words, and actions. The heart-mind stores our experiences, including emotions, in memory, and over time uses this information to construct an identity that defines who we think we are.

Citta is our heart-mind, our outer and inner psyche, and the primary place of interest in the Yoga Sūtras. Our heart-mind sits between the ever-changing outside world and an inner light of awareness. This inner light never changes, and it represents pure, unconditional love. A heart-mind sullied with mental-emotional baggage prevents the inner light from shining through, causing us to act or react according to our deep habitual patterns of behavior. As the heart-mind is clarified, more light can shine through it, and our actions become more loving and positive toward others and ourselves. One of the core aspects of yoga is the process of clarifying the heart-mind (*citta-prasādana*), so external objects are perceived accurately and truthfully.

The *citta* consists of an outer mind, inner mind, ego, and memory. Each component serves a specific purpose, and all of them working together determine how we interact with the world.

Our inner light of awareness (*puruṣa*), resting in stillness, witnesses the operations in the heart-mind. The *puruṣa* illuminates the *citta*, and the *citta* interacts with external objects and events. The *citta* is the middleman between what is outside of us and the *puruṣa*. It is the medium through which perception passes and on which our inner light of awareness shines.

Our *citta* is conditioned during our lifetime. Our personality is based on our innate genetics overlaid by all that we have experienced. Whenever we have an experience, it creates an immediate impression that is stored as a memory in our *citta*. The stronger the impression, the stronger the memory. Over time, these memories program our *citta*, and we develop opinions, biases, prejudices, and habitual behavioral patterns (*saṁskāra-s*) that can make us set in our ways. Our ego is built along the way, giving us healthy self-esteem, insecurity, or an arrogant self-centeredness. Because of this conditioning, each person forms his own unique worldview, so the same object or event may be experienced differently from person to person.

When the *citta* is clear, we perceive objects and events accurately. Exposing ourselves to reliable sources of information (*pramāṇa*) causes truthful memories to be stored. On the other hand, when we believe misleading ideas or outright lies, then our memory can become flawed, even if the *citta* is clear. Positive and truthful memories support similar thoughts and emotions (*vṛtti-s*), while negative, harmful memories contribute to detrimental ones.

All perception and action create impressions in our memory that can affect our subsequent perception and action. Deep patterns cause our *citta* to become biased in one direction or another and distracted by the resulting chatter happening there (*vṛtti-s*). The presence of distracting activities, thoughts, ideas, and baggage is what blocks us from experiencing our inner light of awareness.

The *citta* will be influenced by whatever it is exposed to or focused on. Those around us influence our personality, and vice versa. Being around helpful and positive people who uplift us will provide support and promote happiness, while keeping negative and critical company brings us down. A strong, charismatic personality can compel others to follow, even if it is unhealthy or harmful. For example, many girls will dress like the most popular girl in school. Dressing in any other way may be looked down upon and ridiculed. Conforming to what others deem acceptable is very easy and painless, yet restricts free thinking and individuality for all but the leaders. In college, fraternity brothers will play drinking games that are downright life threatening, just to fit in. Parents serve as models for their children, who spend much of their time following them.

Yoga, because it is focused so much on developing our inner mind rather than keeping up with outer names and forms, is all about independent thinking. Many years of meditation clear and polish our *citta* to the point where our perceptions are clear and our thoughts, words, and deeds are positive and beneficial. Purification and clarification of *citta* (*citta-prasādana*) is the primary result of yoga practice and leads us to connection with our divine inner light of awareness.

It is important to understand what the *citta* is, how it works, and what we can do to refine and clarify it in order to register our experiences truthfully. We can transform our heart-mind field of consciousness by engaging in the practices described in the Yoga Sūtras, such as the eight limbs of yoga. Over time, our communication will improve, and misunderstandings will diminish, leading to more enjoyable social interactions, inner happiness, and a closer connection to our inner light of awareness.

THOUGHTS

The heart-mind is the center of consciousness.

I understand the *citta* as a link between external objects and the inner light of awareness.

I will guide my heart-mind field toward clarity and kindness.

EXERCISES

Think of yourself in broader terms, as if you were a citizen of the world instead of limited to your particular local culture. What might you do differently if you were free to act and not bound by conformity?

Think of times when you changed your mind, replacing what you thought before with something completely different. How did this change affect your worldview? Did you make the change instantly, or did you consider it carefully before making it? Did you make this change as a result of a shift from within or influence from someone or something outside yourself? If someone or something outside yourself convinced you to change your mind, what might that person or thing have to gain by your change of mind?

Which of your habits or behaviors are due to nature (genetic, acting the way your parents acted when they were your age) and which are due to nurture (based on your life experience)?

3

PURUṢA

Pure Inner Light of Awareness

पुरुष

Weapons cannot cut this, fire cannot burn this,
water cannot wet this, nor can wind make it dry.
BHAGAVAD GĪTĀ 2.23

SEATED IN OUR HEART AND pervading every cell of our body lies a conscious, intelligent awareness. Individual uniqueness is due to our temporary, ever-changing body, breath, and mind. These outer layers of ourselves surround an inner, divine light of awareness called the *puruṣa* or *ātman*, which illuminates the truth and expresses love and compassion.

Our thoughts and emotions can distort what we perceive, creating in our heart-mind a cloud that blurs what we register in memory. The process of yoga includes practices to quiet down and clarify our heart-mind so that this inner essence can shed light on whatever we experience and reveal what is true and actual.

Puruṣa is difficult to explain in words or understand intellectually. The rational mind has trouble grasping anything that cannot be perceived by the sensory organs or cannot be constructed based on logic and/or hard evidence. Sometimes unanswerable questions, like the koans of Zen Buddhism, serve to shock the logical mind and wake us up to new possibilities. For example, "what is the sound of one hand clapping?" As we turn our attention inward through introspection and meditation (*saṁyama*), the rational mind softens and opens, allowing indescribable experiences to occur. Like the taste of honey, some things can only be known through experience.

Most religions celebrate and revere a divinity. Many ancient texts, poems, and songs from various cultures around the world express devotion to the divine. Often the experience of connection with the divine is so inexplicable that metaphor is required just to get an inkling. Nihilism, where the divine is described as not this, not that, not anything that words can convey, is a common technique as well. On the other hand, yoga primarily addresses how we can experience this pure inner awareness.

This divine inner spectator, also called the seer, simply watches events unfold in the heart-mind. It sees only what the heart-mind presents to it. The *puruṣa* provides the light that shines through the moment-by-moment frames in the heart-mind, projecting our personality out onto the screen of the world.

The *puruṣa* is the individual spirit that is part of a universal spirit. The greeting *namaste* literally means "salutations to you." On a deeper level, it connotes honoring the *puruṣa* that resides inside another person. Seeing all beings as manifestations of the same light of awareness allows us to detach from outer labels, opinions, and judgments and to act in a kinder and more compassionate way. Humans look different on the outside, but our basic, inner nature is the same. The realization that all life forms share the same inner consciousness encourages us to act toward others as if they are ourselves.

It may be easier to understand *puruṣa* in terms of what it is not: the material world (*dṛśya* or *prakṛti*), matter and energy, which are considered unconscious and transient. *Puruṣa* is the underlying consciousness that pervades every atom of the manifest world, yet is not affected by any of its changes. This background seer can influence our heart-mind by its loving presence alone. In fact, one goal of practicing yoga is to reach the state in which our decisions and actions are based on perceiving our environment clearly and accurately, illumined by the inner light of awareness, as opposed to functioning with clouded perception, induced by our ego to think we are nothing but the chatter and habitual patterns active in our heart-mind.

The *puruṣa*—quiet, still, and changeless—watches the activities present in our heart-mind. Have you ever noticed how when we become quiet and still, whatever is happening around us becomes much clearer and easier to observe? For example, if you walk through a mall while talking to a friend, you will notice much, much less than you would if you were sitting on a bench, watching everything go on. Sitting down in a forest reveals so much more activity than hiking and/or talking within the forest. Slowing down our pace in life reduces stress and enables us to observe the outside world much more clearly. Calming our breath and nervous system (*prāṇāyāma*) and clarifying our heart-mind (*citta-prasādana*) will improve communication and social interactions. For example, taking a deep breath or sighing heavily automatically relaxes and slows you down, allowing you to take a quiet moment for yourself before you make an important decision.

Underneath our changing body, breath, thoughts, and emotions lies a softly glowing light of awareness. The tools and techniques provided by Patañjali in the Yoga Sūtras are all meant to clear our heart and mind for the single purpose of connecting with this *puruṣa*. Along the way, these practices reduce impurities, cultivate inner contentment, and cause us to become kind and compassionate citizens of the world by enabling us to see this divine essence within all sentient beings.

THOUGHTS

There is an unchanging, pure awareness
that illuminates my consciousness

I can catch glimpses of this inner light by quieting
my heart-mind and focusing inward.

I will practice yoga to clarify my heart-mind and
allow the light of awareness to shine through.

EXERCISES

Meditate on the part of you that never changes.

How does a belief in a divine entity help people
cope with the ups and downs of life?

Sit quietly and ponder why the vast majority of the
world's population believes in some higher power, even
as more and more mysteries are explained by science.

4

DṚŚYA

Ever-Changing Mother Nature

दृश्य

Listen
all creeping things—
the bell of transience.
ISSA

THE WORLDVIEW OF YOGA INCLUDES the belief that all material substances are in a constant state of flux. Modern science, especially atomic and quantum theory, agrees. Even our DNA mutates slowly every moment. Understanding the transitory nature of all things is prerequisite to letting go of expectations and attachments. Our senses interact with the outer world, yet we have the potential to turn our attention inward and experience that which never changes, our inner light of awareness (*puruṣa*).

Dṛśya, meaning "what is seeable," is what the seer witnesses—the entire cosmic process; all matter and energy that encompass the changing, manifest world; everything but the seer. Synonyms for *dṛśya* are *prakṛti*, meaning "nature," and *māyā*, meaning "measurable, illusion."

The material, manifest world as a whole is considered to be feminine, as in Mother Nature. Other English words related to mother are *matter* and *matrix*, each describing different characteristics of the observable universe. All of these words derive from the Sanskrit word for mother, *mātṛ*. In this context, the father correlates to the *puruṣa*, the seer, which pervades the universe without being affected by its changes.

SEER (*Draṣṭṛ/Puruṣa*)	SEEABLE (*Dṛśya/Prakṛti*)
conscious	unconscious
inactive	active
permanent	impermanent
intelligent	unintelligent
unchanging	changing
unmanifest	manifest
observer	observable
subject	object
independent	dependent
uniform	composite

The seer (*puruṣa*), the instrument of seeing (*citta*), and the seen (*dṛśya*) all play their parts during perception. Imagine that the seer is sitting quietly in its own luminosity, watching from behind the scenes. It sees the outside world through the heart-mind (*citta*), the middleman. If the *citta* is clear and quiet, then the seer sees the world as it actually is, and its light is able to shine out into the world for the benefit of all. On the other hand, if our *citta* is busy, then distracting thoughts and emotions (*vṛtti-s*) create interference, like white noise from an improper television signal. Instead of seeing the world clearly, the seer observes distortion and confusion.

Distinguishing between the seer and the seen is a major realization that is said to remove the dark covering of ignorance (*avidyā*) in the heart-mind, allowing the light of the seer to illumine our heart-mind, which finally experiences its true nature. Thinking the seer and seeable are the same (*saṁyoga*) is the basic blunder that prevents us from connecting with our inner light of awareness.

Enlightenment (*kaivalya*) occurs when the heart-mind is totally clarified and purified of all possible negativity and causes of suffering. Such rare, enlightened people radiate unconditional love and acceptance. The pure light of the seer can shine through their eyes completely. Looking at them (*darśana*) is like looking into a clear mirror of the soul, in which we can see ourselves reflected exactly as we are, not as we think we are.

The world around us is not the same as it was a moment ago, and its changes are not always predictable. When our expectations are not met or a sudden tragedy befalls us, we can move on more easily when we understand the temporality of ourselves and our surroundings. The seer within is our only rock, and connecting our consciousness to it can ground us and carry us through all matter of events and experiences.

THOUGHTS

A conscious, permanent, inner light of awareness
pervades the impermanent, changing universe.

I can alleviate suffering by distinguishing between
what changes and what never changes.

I will begin to accept the transient nature of all things
by the persistent and sincere practice of yoga.

Exercises

The next time you go to a movie in a theater, imagine the blank screen is your *citta*; the images projected on the screen are your thoughts, emotions, and perceptions, and the light that allows you to see the images is the seer within you. Think about the illusory, changing nature of the images. Notice, too, the emptiness, clarity, and brightness that arises when there are no images in the way.

The next time your expectations are not met, see if you become upset. Explore what you were or are attached to that caused the upset, and then view that thing as yet another changing entity within your seeable world.

Each time you see an object that looks like it does not change, such as a rock, think about how it might have become what it is, and what it might change to in a thousand or a million years.

5

VIVEKA

Keen Discernment

विवेक

Sometimes the questions are complicated
and the answers are simple.
DR. SEUSS

THE ABILITY TO CHOOSE WISELY and separate the wheat from the chaff is fundamental to the practice of yoga. Without this ability, our thoughts, words, and actions are limited to the whim of habitual tendency and the prison of involuntary conformity. Yoga involves a commitment to freeing our heart and mind of unnecessary and unhelpful baggage and focusing instead on our path toward contentment and inner happiness.

Viveka is knowing and consciously discerning one object from another. We are making decisions and judgments all the time, every day, such as what to eat, how to dress, where to go, and what to do. Exercising clear judgment, taking into account what is helpful versus harmful and what works in the short term versus the long term, can help us avoid future suffering. Access to as much information as possible gives us the broadest view and highest chance of making the best decision.

For example, you are interviewing people for positions at your company. It is up to you to determine the most important characteristics you are looking for, beyond just qualifications on paper. Someone who may not have much experience but learns quickly and is thorough might fare better than one who has so much experience that they are set in their ways and cannot adapt easily. Sometimes the simple quality of getting along with others is more important than anything else. *Viveka* is all the more important if you are hiring someone for a long-term position.

Viveka helps us make healthy choices in life. Stepping back and quietly contemplating what we really want in life can initiate actions in that direction. What kind of career do we want? What qualities are we looking for in a life partner? Which places would we like to live in or explore? Using keen discernment, we can carve for ourselves a path that is happier and more fulfilling. The choices we make now determine our future.

In any action, it is important to know who or where we are now (our current state), where we want to go (a direction), and the steps necessary to get there. Observing ourselves closely, through quiet contemplation, and listening to others can give us a sense of who we are. How we react to touchy situations can provide valuable information about our deep behavioral patterns. Recognizing the existence of our discomfort or pain (*duḥkha*), identifying its cause, and then working to consciously weaken that cause will eventually eliminate suffering. Keen discernment along the way is not only helpful but also necessary for this process to be effective.

Viveka can help us avoid being harmed due to lack of knowledge or experience. For example, a child may see a colorful mushroom as something that might taste good, unaware it is toxic, while a botanist or mycologist could discern the difference between an edible and a poisonous mushroom.

Viveka also means separating what is useful from what is not, like throwing away the inedible outer peel of an orange and keeping the juicy inner part. We can minimize contact with those who bring us down and influence us in a harmful way, while maximizing our time spent in the company of people who support our chosen path. We may have teachers who are filled with wisdom, yet falter in other areas of life. We can listen to and integrate the wisdom while not allowing their failings to affect us.

On a deeper, internal level, *viveka* can help us distinguish between our changing body and our unchanging inner light of awareness. Without *viveka*, individuals identify the body as themselves—they think they are their body and nothing more. With *viveka*, the body is seen as an instrument only, a formation of matter and energy that does not affect our true nature, our inner light of awareness.

Keen discernment results from practicing the eight limbs of yoga (*aṣṭāṅga*), which remove impurities from the body and clear the heart-mind of undesirable baggage, allowing the inner light of awareness to shine through. Whenever our faculty of judgment listens to our clear, inner voice instead of our ego, we act selflessly.

Viveka supports diligent practice (*abhyāsa*) and not clinging to external objects (*vairāgya*). As we learn to step back and quietly observe what is going on around us, we can figure out what action would be most beneficial to ourselves and others at the same time. As we observe our own personal practice, we can carefully discern what is working and what is not, and then make modifications to maximize our efforts. As we turn inward, more and more outer objects and events become useless to us and we are able to let go of any attachment to them.

THOUGHTS

Distinguishing what changes from the unchanging light within us is a way to end suffering.

With a clear heart-mind, I can develop the ability to determine what is helpful and what is not.

I will make wise and informed decisions for the benefit of all sentient beings.

EXERCISES

The next time you have to make an important decision, collect as much information as possible, then sit quietly for some time. Try and view all the angles before making your decision. Will peer pressure factor into your decision?

When you see someone whom you need to interact with, but do not like very much, try and separate their personality from the divine inner light of awareness residing within them. Take time to meditate on the dynamic between you, and see if there is a way to improve your interactions.

Think of areas in your life where you could practice more *viveka* and how you might practice it.

6

ABHYĀSA

Diligent, Focused Practice

अभ्यास

Be soft in your practice. Think of the method as a fine silvery stream, not a raging waterfall. Follow the stream, have faith in its course. It will go on its own way, meandering here, trickling there. It will find the grooves, the cracks, the crevices. Just follow it. Never let it out of your sight. It will take you.

SHENG YEN

MAKING PROGRESS IN ANY ENDEAVOR requires time, effort, and focus. World-class athletes develop their prowess after many years of continuous practice. What we learn from teachers and books is important, yet secondary to the knowledge we acquire through direct experience. That which cannot be described in words and can only be alluded to, the knowledge of our inner Self (*puruṣa*), absolutely requires turning our attention inward on a regular basis.

Abhyāsa is a disciplined, persistent effort to remain focused. This focus can occur during physical exercise (such as *āsana*), breath work (*prāṇāyāma*), meditation (*saṁyama*), or even the act of learning a musical instrument or driving a car. The *sūtra-s* state that *abhyāsa* is the effort required to maintain a focus, and it is to be done continuously over a long period of time, with sincerity and care. *Abhyāsa* involves a committed effort to maintain your chosen practice long enough to reap its rewards. *Abhyāsa*, along with *viveka* (keen discernment), is a primary practice that is fundamental to all progress.

If we want to acquire a new skill and become proficient at it, training over time is necessary. Going to an institute of learning, such as a university or trade school, provides the structure, duration, and teaching required to achieve our goal. Continuing education is helpful for keeping our skills up-to-date. *Abhyāsa* brings us to a professional level of performance, providing us with the knowledge and expertise to acquire a better job and even teach others.

Abhyāsa can also apply to understanding another person. Focusing on that person regularly over time, with sincerity and respect, allows us to truly understand her better. Understanding others helps us understand parts of ourselves. For example, a close family member is hard to be around. You create a "practice" with the purpose of improving your relationship with her. Let's say your mother is always giving you unsolicited advice. Your practice might be to understand that, for some reason, she feels the need to mother you, even though you are a grown adult who is doing fine on your own. Allowing her to mother may make her feel needed in some way, yet enabling that behavior may not serve you in the end. One way or another, it is important to think of a way for you and her to be able to interact that satisfies her and does not get under your skin.

Abhyāsa, along with not clinging to external objects (*vairāgya*), is necessary to calm down the heart-mind (*yoga as nirodha*). Consistent and persistent effort, along with the ability to not let external events throw us off center, is bound to diminish the thoughts and emotions distracting our heart-mind. In the classical sense, there is no yoga practice without *abhyāsa* and *vairāgya*.

In the beginning, it can be difficult to establish a regular practice. *Abhyāsa* can prevent or counteract certain obstacles to yoga (*antarāya-s*), such as disease, doubt, and apathy. Diligent, focused practice will reduce or eliminate their detrimental effects. Each time we practice, an impression is made in our subconscious heart-mind. Over time, the *abhyāsa* becomes a habit (*saṁskāra*) that eventually becomes stronger than other, less helpful habits. As the momentum of this *abhyāsa* strengthens, practicing becomes easier, and the beneficial results accrue.

For example, we want to learn how to cook our own meals instead of eating at restaurants all the time. At first, it takes a while to acquire the ingredients and follow the recipes. Each time we make the same dishes, they become easier. Eventually, the recipes that began as difficult and time consuming seem fast and simple. For another example, if you come down with a disease that is hard to shake, establishing healthy dietary, exercise, and lifestyle habits can help you overcome this obstacle and move in a positive and hopeful direction.

It is important to stay on track and not give up, even when we want to. Practice makes perfect. If we can get ourselves into a good routine, practicing becomes habitual and, thus, easier. Whether we attend regular *āsana* classes or set aside time every morning to sit quietly and meditate, perseverance will ensure some level of progress. Over time, our body, breath, heart, and mind will become more clear, refined, and pure, benefiting not only ourselves but everyone around us as well.

THOUGHTS

Ongoing, sincere, and effortful practice is the source of my strength and progress.

Consistent, focused practice will diminish distractions, reduce attachment to superficial matters, and deepen the connection to my divine inner Self.

Every time I practice, it empowers me and reinforces my positive direction.

EXERCISES

If you do not yet have a regular practice, carve out some time in your day, even if it is only ten minutes, to spend connecting with your inner Self. Make this practice a priority, even higher than checking your email or answering the telephone.

If you already have a regular practice, focus your mind on only the practice, not allowing it to wander as your practice becomes too familiar and rote. You can also focus your mind during any regular activity, such as cooking or cleaning.

If you have a difficult person in your life, perhaps a relative, a neighbor, or a coworker, how can you practice improving your interactions with them? Come up with a few concrete ideas, and notice what happens when you implement them.

7

VAIRĀGYA

Nonattachment to Sensory Objects

वैराग्य

The secret of happiness lies
in the mind's release from worldly ties.
THE BUDDHA

WHEN OUR ATTENTION IS DRAWN outward, our heart-mind becomes entangled in the complex net of everyday activity. Attachments to things develop, until we are so involved with them that we lose perspective, identifying ourselves in terms of outer names and forms. As we slow down and turn inward, connecting with our inner light of awareness that quietly watches everything happening, we naturally lose interest in external, transient objects. We realize that the ups and downs of life come and go, ever spinning around the motionless hub of *puruṣa*.

Vairāgya is characterized by an indifference to objects and a detachment from them. When an object is perceived, it can produce an attraction, which can lead to an attachment. Over time the attachment may grow into a craving, and not experiencing the object again will upset us. If we are unaffected by the presence or absence of something, then *vairāgya* is happening. For example, you climbed to the top of the corporate ladder and became attached to the power, control, and money that came with it. Then the company was bought out, and you lost your position. If you had become attached to the image of yourself as powerful, you might feel lost at sea without your job. But if you were able to do your job without attaching your identity to it, you will experience this change without anxiety or fear.

Actions repeated over and over create deep habitual patterns (*saṁskara-s*) in our consciousness and usually influence future action. *Vairāgya* is to not allow our past action patterns, addictions, or strong desires to affect our focus. Diligent practice (*abhyāsa*) directed inward will, over time, cultivate *vairāgya*. For example, as you meditate regularly and reach the point at which you feel connected to that ever-present divine light of awareness, you want to stay there as long as possible. When your attention returns to the outer world, things that you now know are temporary do not seem to matter as much. Your priorities may shift. If you are approaching old age and have accumulated a lot of money, you may realize that you will be happier by letting some of that go to those who really need it.

Consciously directing our desires inward is different than attempting to restrict our outer desires. Wants and needs are part of living in a society—we cannot live without them. It is natural to desire and enjoy being around people you care about, to be attracted to beautiful things, or even to have fun with the latest electronic gadget. There is nothing inherently wrong with desiring something. Artificially withholding from ourselves goes against the natural flow of life and is not *vairāgya*. But if we cannot fulfill our desires, if we cannot have what we want, do we become angry or frustrated? If so, then we are attached to those desires, and therefore, psychologically bound by them.

Vairāgya is in place when we are OK either way, whether or not our desires are satisfied. The inner contentment that grows from connecting to our inner light of awareness makes us not care as much about outer desires. When our primary desire is to experience the divinity within, then external objects lose their appeal.

The process of *vairāgya* occurs in stages. First, we identify an attachment by observing how we are (*svādhyāya*) when we do not get what we want. If we are thrown off center, then attachment is there. Next, we play with the attachment by occasionally not fulfilling the desire for it. Next, over time, we notice ourselves detached from the weaker attachments, but still connected to the stronger ones. Eventually, even the strong attachments go away, and we lose our desire for them. In the final stage, we tackle internal attachments, such as our reputation (*asmitā-kleśa*), aversions (*dveṣa-kleśa-s*), and habits (*saṁskāra-s*).

Another school of thought outlines the steps leading up to the state of *vairāgya*. First, as our desire turns inward, outer desires become less tempting. Over time, we naturally develop an attitude of nonattachment. Then the sensory organs become detached from objects, but the tendency for attachment remains in the mind. Eventually, there is no more effort or conflict, and desire for the object has gone away.

Vairāgya and *abhyāsa* are necessary for quieting any distracting thoughts and emotions (*yoga as nirodha*). Both are considered pillars of yoga that, with *viveka*, form the backbone of yoga practice. During meditation, *abhyāsa* is the effort exerted to stay on the point of focus, while *vairāgya* pulls our wandering attention back to the focus. For example, let's say you are meditating. You begin to focus on your chosen object. After a few seconds or minutes, those pesky little *vṛtti-s* distract you and carry your attention elsewhere. At some point, you become aware that you are in *vṛtti* land and bring yourself back to the focus. This awareness can be considered *vairāgya*.

Vairāgya is not a struggle with desires, but the result of an enduring *abhyāsa* that naturally leads to a disinclination toward worldly desires. The goal is to keep our heart-mind focused on the inner light of awareness that is inside of us and all other sentient beings. The more our attention is there, the happier we are. Letting go of outer attachments unloads a burden that is weighing us down and keeping us from experiencing the freedom that is yoga.

THOUGHTS

Attachment to that which inevitably changes causes suffering.

As my heart-mind turns inward, I become less and less affected by external objects and conditions.

I will be deeply content when I do not depend on material things to make me happy.

EXERCISES

Think of situations in which remaining indifferent is helpful to yourself and others. Are you able to be that way? Why or why not? Identify possible attachments associated with the situation. How can you detach from them?

As you establish an *abhyāsa* practice, notice what attachments naturally fade. For example, when you begin doing regular aerobic exercise to replace idle time, you may notice yourself daydreaming less. Or if you start a vigorous *āsana* practice, a high libido may adjust to normal as you feel your body stretching and moving.

Sit quietly and meditate. Notice the path of your attention as it moves toward and away from the point of focus. Making a list of your to-dos beforehand may help reduce the amount of time your mind wanders.

8

YOGA AS NIRODHA

Silencing the Heart-Mind

योग निरोध

Love opens my chest, and thought
returns to its confines.
RUMI, from GRANITE AND WINEGLASS

DURING THE JOURNEY THROUGH LIFE, our heart-mind (*citta*) accumulates memories from every experience, which influence our thoughts, emotions, and, therefore, our actions. The activities buzzing around in our consciousness make us think that we are these actions. Yoga is, by definition, a process of quieting these activities in order to be able to look deeply within and connect with that which never moves, our divine inner light of awareness (*puruṣa*).

Yoga is defined in the second *sūtra* as a process of thinning away or quieting (*nirodha*) the thoughts and emotions in our heart-mind. *Nirodha* results from the practices of yoga, especially a focused heart-mind. *Nirodha* is not actively avoiding, suspending, or ending our thoughts and emotions. Rather it occurs naturally when our attention is focused in one direction, causing those distractions to submerge and the inner light of knowledge to emerge.

As a process or practice, yoga is connecting our individual consciousness to the universal consciousness. Several yoga practices are mentioned in Patañjali's *sūtra-s.* The eight limbs of yoga (*aṣṭāṅga*) provide tools to refine ourselves and draw our attention inward. *Kriyā-yoga,* the synergistic triad composed of transformational practice, self-observation, and faith, is meant to weaken our deep afflictions and attain a state of complete attention (*samādhi*). We could say that *saṁyama-yoga* (the final three inner limbs) expresses a subset of the eight limbs that represents focusing inward and experiencing *samādhi.*

Yoga can also be a state equivalent to *samādhi* resulting from the process of *nirodha.* When we are in the state of yoga, our consciousness is quiet, and we experience the presence of our inner light of awareness, our true Self. *Yoga* means "union" or "connection" with this divine presence. This seer (*puruṣa*) is resting in the perception of itself and is experienced as clarity, understanding, compassion, and happiness. In this state, our attention is so focused that the activities (*vṛtti-s*) in the heart-mind no longer distract us. Our field of consciousness has absorbed whatever it is focused on so completely that we cannot perceive any difference between it and us. We are unaware of our awareness because there is no separation between our individual self and our inner Self. Until this state is present, we are in *vṛtti* land, preoccupied, caught in the world of thoughts and memories, where our individual ego erroneously identifies us as our *vṛtti-s.*

Certain states of mind lead us through the process of *nirodha.* At first, the *citta* is restless and rapid, which can cause delusion, infatuation, or obsession. Our thoughts are moving so fast, and we are so caught up in them, that it is difficult to perceive the outer world clearly. As we spend more time cultivating inner peace, our *citta* alternates between calmness and restlessness. Over time, our *citta* becomes one pointed, able to focus on a single thought continuously. Eventually, this leads to the state of yoga, where the heart-mind is still, undistracted by any thoughts, emotions, or sensory input.

Nirodha depends on two pillars of yoga: *abhyāsa* and *vairāgya.* The former, diligent and continuous practice, results in the latter, detached awareness, which, in turn, causes *nirodha.* As the busyness in the heart-mind slows down, the fluctuations become simpler and less distracting. As *nirodha* is practiced regularly over time, the fluctuations erode, and a new, beneficial pattern forms to eventually supersede previous, negative tendencies. This reprogramming of the heart-mind is the key to inner happiness.

Stress can occur when our heart-mind is overwhelmed with activity or emotion. There are simple ways to reduce or prevent stress. Many people become stressed-out when they are running late for an appointment, often the result of not leaving enough time to get where they're going. It is easy enough to instead anticipate the time required to make it on time, prepare for the appointment early, and then allow an extra buffer of time to avoid becoming stressed. In the likely event you make it there early, you can enjoy the wait by sitting quietly and relaxing.

Yoga is both the process of quieting and the state of quiescence. Consciously tuning out any distracting noise around us and turning our attention inward nurtures our heart and mind. Slowing down and connecting with our silent inner light of awareness relieves us from the hustle and bustle of the world.

THOUGHTS

Directing my attention inward on a regular basis
will cause distracting thoughts to subside and
allow my inner light to shine through.

A quiet, calm heart-mind enables me to see things clearly
and make wise choices that benefit myself and others.

I will cultivate a clear and open heart-mind.

EXERCISES

How effective has your yoga practice been for
calming down your mind? Try spending a little less
time on the postures and a little more time sitting
quietly and turning your attention inward.

Think about what situations make you restless, such as leaving at the last minute and rushing to an appointment, or doing so many things at once that your head seems to spin. Then think of ways you can prevent these situations from happening, like leaving early to an appointment or scaling back your schedule.

Use an everyday activity to practice one-pointedness.
For example, when you brush your teeth, work on your
computer, or prepare a meal, do so with one-pointed
attention. Do this exercise for a week, and notice
how your relationship to the activity changes.

9

ĪŚVARA

The Source of Knowledge

ईश्वर

Spirituality dawns when the intellect is silenced
by loving devotion and reverential humility.
KIRPAL SINGH

SCIENCE, PHILOSOPHY, AND RELIGION often overlap, and yoga involves all three. It is a science because it presents knowledge of the physical world based on observation and experience. As a philosophy, it investigates truth and principles of existence, knowledge, and conduct. Finally, since yoga describes matters of a very fine and subtle nature, and is based on a theory of creation that involves an unchanging, permanent, divine awareness (*puruṣa*), it has a religious aspect as well.

Īśvara is described in the *sūtra-s* as a kind of *puruṣa*. Whereas *puruṣa* is the individual soul embedded in our body and exposed to the activities occurring in our heart-mind, *īśvara* is its universal correlate, unbound and untouched by anything at all. While our individual *puruṣa* watches and is entertained by the manifest dance of *prakṛti*, *īśvara* simply exists.

Īśvara is the pure light of knowledge, the macrocosmic energy of omniscience that we tap into through our inner light of knowledge and awareness (*puruṣa*). Although it is conscious of all actions, it cannot act, but can influence action. Actions coming from the place of *īśvara* create beneficial (yogic) behavioral patterns (*saṁskāra-s*). In any given situation, a broader, more informed heart-mind allows us to see the whole picture, understand all points of view, and then act for the benefit of everyone. For example, a general contractor who has years of experience and a wide range of knowledge can anticipate and avoid potential pitfalls that a novice would otherwise fall into.

Īśvara is also considered a teacher, and it can bring about transformation just as a human teacher can catalyze inspiration and insight in a student's heart-mind by the transmission of knowledge. The *sūtra-s* state that *īśvara* is the original and eternal teacher, not limited by time. All knowledge learned in the manifest world ultimately sprouts from the seed of *īśvara*. This universal intelligence always was, is, and will be available to those who seek to understand the truth.

Believing in something greater than ourselves cultivates humility. One way to prevent egotism (*asmitā*) is to think of *īśvara* as all knowledge that ever existed or will ever exist. Then, whenever we come up with a new idea or create something unique, instead of believing it is ours to patent or exclusively use to promote our own self-interest, we can think of it as tapping into a bank of knowledge that was there all along. In ancient India, authors rarely ascribed their name to the books they wrote. They saw themselves as simply presenting what they learned from their teachers and life experience in a more understandable way, participating in the ongoing transmission of knowledge that belongs to no one. Surrendering and transferring the results of all action to *īśvara* (*īśvara-praṇidhāna*) is a powerful practice that can keep us from thinking we are better than anyone else.

Many cultures and religions talk about creation beginning with sound or light. Patañjali says that this original sound is a direct expression of *īśvara* and, therefore, provides a direct link to it. In India's ancient tradition of yoga, this sound is *Om*. *Īśvara* is in a sense the meaning of *Om*, and by saying or chanting *Om*, we are able to connect to this divine source of knowledge. *Om* is the genesis of creation, and its sound is not random. *Om* is made of three sounds: *a*, *u*, and *m*. In Sanskrit, *a* plus *u* always combine to form *o*. *A* is made in the very beginning of the mouth, at the back of the throat, and *u* is made at the very end of the mouth, at the lips. So the sound itself causes vibration to span the entire mouth, which symbolizes all of creation. The final *m* creates a hum that drives the *o* into our body.

A mantra is simply a sound that has a specific effect, which becomes stronger as it is recited over and over again. The more something is repeated, the more powerful its effect on our consciousness is. Repeating *Om* links our consciousness to *īśvara* and allows us to feel its essence. Repeating *Om* also draws our attention inward and causes outer distractions to disappear. Sound has a way of reprogramming the consciousness and dissolving obstacles (*antarāya-s*), like disease and doubt.

Īśvara can be worshipped through a personal source of devotion, a symbol that links us to it. This source can be a spiritual teacher, a sacred text, a diety, or even science itself. In India's Hindu religion, there are many interesting deities to choose from. One that is broadly accepted as a universally positive symbol is Gaṇeśa, the elephant-headed deity representing abundance and the clearing away of obstacles.

Belief in *īśvara* implies that we have faith in a divine intelligence, a whole that is greater than our individual self. The endless macrocosm's universality will always reflect the individuality of our limited microcosm. Connecting and synchronizing with the greater community, nation, world, and universe will keep us living in tune with the rhythms of nature.

THOUGHTS

I deeply respect the divine energy untouched
by the ever-changing world around me.

I can connect to the pure inner light of knowledge
by uttering the sacred sound of creation.

I will endeavor to make informed decisions
and understand all points of view.

EXERCISES

Think of a symbol that represents *īśvara* to you,
such as a prophet, deity, or even a religion. Sit
quietly and meditate on this symbol.

Find out what sound began creation according to
whatever religion you practice. If there is none, try
using *Om* by chanting it over and over again, thereby
linking to this universal light of knowledge.

Think of the teachers who have influenced you
most in your life. Sit quietly and pay homage to

them, thanking them for passing on such valuable knowledge. They are each a form of *īśvara* for you.

10

KARMA AND SAṀSKĀRA

Action and Its Imprint

कर्म संस्कार

Do unto others as you would have them do unto you.
LUKE 6:31

KARMA IS A POPULAR WORD with many connotations. *Karma* means action or activity that produces a result and leaves behind an energetic impression inside our heart-mind. *Karma* can originate from us as a thought, word, or deed, or it can be something we perceive with our senses, such as a movie we watch or song that we hear. Every *karma* has consequences, which may occur sooner or later and may be obvious or subtle. *Karma* is recorded in our memory and, it is said, in the memory bank of the universe.

On a cosmic level, Isaac Newton's third law of motion states, "For every action, there is an equal and opposite reaction." The cause of an action contains its effects in subtle form. The universe is a continuous dance of energy. If we want to contribute the energy of kindness and compassion to the universe, we must act that way. Positive energy begets positive energy, and vice versa. For example, have you noticed how you feel around someone who is kind, generous, and happy? Does it make you feel more that way? On the other hand, when you are in the company of a negative, mean, pessimistic person, how do you feel? Our heart-mind (*citta*) influences and is influenced by whatever we choose to be around.

Karma has the sense of retribution. It is said, "What goes around comes around." On an individual level, the science of yoga accepts the theory of reincarnation, where an individual soul inhabits body after body through cycles of birth and death. The soul is said to carry the residue of our actions from life to life, seeking to improve each time. If a person evolves spiritually and acts in a virtuous way, without being attached to the results, then these actions do not accumulate in memory. Eventually, the previously incurred *karma* works itself out, and the person is said to become enlightened (*kaivalya*), never to be reborn again. On the other hand, if individuals degrade over the course of their lifetime, then it is said they will be reborn into a more difficult life, maybe even as a lower form of consciousness, such as a snake or insect. Therefore, the law of *karma* encourages us to act selflessly and for the benefit of others.

It may take a long time, even another lifetime, for karmic payback to happen. Each time you perform a positive action, it is like depositing money into your karmic bank account. Each time you do something hurtful or negative, it is like writing a check from that bank account. The goal is to build up as much karmic currency as possible in order to ensure your current and future lifetimes will be filled with positive, happy energy. The bottom line is the golden rule: whatever effects our actions have, those effects will come back to us at some point in the future.

According to yoga, actions can be good, bad, or neutral, and each type will create impressions in memory accordingly. These actions are often influenced or directed by our deep conditioning and so are considered to be somewhat unconscious, programmed by our past.

In addition to action, there are inaction and nonaction, and each has different results. Inaction is the gray limbo of indecision, when we cannot decide what to do. This is considered the worst form of action because nothing is moving or happening. It is said in business that even a bad decision is better than no decision at all. Arjuna, the protagonist in the Bhagavad Gītā, represents a human who is caught in this stifling state of mind. Kṛṣṇa, his divine counselor, encourages him to act even though that action appears on the outside to go against what seems right. Inaction goes against the flow of the universe, which is moving and changing all the time.

Nonaction is the eventual goal—acting directly from our unconditioned, pure inner Self, with no attachment to the results. This kind of action is not directed or influenced by our conditioning (*saṁskāra-s*). We are not really the doer and, thus, do not create any new or reinforce any existing *saṁskāra-s*. Nonaction means acting selflessly and offering the results to the divine. Voluntarily feeding the hungry at a soup kitchen and considering every serving of food to be an offering to the universe is an example of nonaction. The actions of a true yogin are considered nonactions, which, because they are selfless and serve to weaken distracting *saṁskāra-s*, move the yogin closer to a heart-mind connected to pure awareness.

Every time we register an event (receive a sensory input or produce a thought, word, or deed), a subtle impression is recorded in our memory. The more intense the event or the more it is repeated, the stronger the impression. Eventually, the impression forms a deep imprint, called a *saṁskāra*, which becomes part of who we are and influences our actions. For example, glancing at a squirrel on the road for a split second will leave a relatively weak impression. Going through a painful, traumatic experience, such as a car crash, will create a much stronger impression that may change how we drive in the future. These deep impressions form habits, tendencies, and proclivities that affect the way we think and act.

Negative or harmful *saṁskāra-s* can strengthen the *kleśa-s*, our deepest afflictions and causes of suffering. When our buttons get pushed, an event has triggered these hurtful parts of ourselves, which then arise from the depths of our memory and cause us to react in a negative way. For example, let's say you have sat in the same chair at the kitchen table for the past twenty years. If your son visits and sits in "your" chair for dinner, you may feel uncomfortable, and you may become a little flustered at first. You might become angry and demand that your son sit in another chair. Or you may ask him politely to sit elsewhere. Either way, there is an underlying *saṁskāra* affecting your behavior, one that has been reinforced for many years, even though, on the outside, it seems quite trivial.

Saṁskāra-s can be habits or even addictions. For example, the more you exercise, the more habitual it becomes. As momentum builds, it gets easier and takes less effort to get up and go. But while this type of conscious change moves us in our intended direction, unconscious change may hinder our path. If you stop exercising for a while, the habit weakens, possibly to be replaced by something else you begin doing more often. When exercise is relegated to the back burner, your body gradually weakens. This process can be applied to manipulating our own heart-mind toward yoga. For example, you notice yourself criticizing others without even thinking about it. You want to become less critical and more understanding, so you set an intention to do so. Every time you notice yourself actively criticizing someone, you immediately stop yourself and replace your criticism with kind, constructive words. Over time, as you criticize less and speak positively more often, the harmful habit will fade as the helpful habit strengthens.

Saṁskāra-s can set us in our ways and make us think that everyone should live and behave as we do. If we encounter people who go against our ingrained way of thinking, we may judge them unfairly, deeming them weird, unusual, or even malevolent. For example, you grow up surrounded by people who believe that modern medicine is the best system of medicine for all conditions, and no other system of healing is valid. Whenever you go to doctors, you naturally assume they know literally everything there is to know about disease and its treatment. When you encounter alternative healers, you immediately write them off as quacks, thus generating negative energy toward them. Later on in your life, you become aware of other healing modalities that have worked for your friends when modern medicine did not. Yoga is about opening ourselves to improvement and new ideas, rather than remaining stuck in the closed loops of deep subconscious patterns.

In the modern science of neurobiology, the study of the brain, there are two sayings: "Use it or lose it" and "Neurons that fire together wire together." Whatever thoughts or emotions we experience on a regular basis remain available to us in our heart-mind. If we divert our attention from certain thoughts or emotions, they will gradually become "lost." Therefore, negative *saṁskāra-s* will naturally weaken when our attention is elsewhere. The second saying supports the idea of how a *saṁskāra* forms in the first place. When an action is repeated over and over again, the neurons involved become more and more wired together as their connection is reinforced. The stronger the wiring, the more the resulting behavioral pattern will influence our actions.

Saṁskāra-s can be ended by discovering what caused them. Tracing back a pattern to its origin (*pratiprasava*) allows us to understand how it began and then take steps toward minimizing its influence on our future actions. Taking these steps requires effort and a deep willingness to improve ourselves and our actions.

Understanding what *karma* and *saṁskāra* are and how they work together is fundamental to fully comprehending yoga itself. Every single thought, word, deed, and impression affects us in some way. Working toward the goal of making our actions positive and helpful, all the time, will make us and those around us happier and healthier, and move us closer to experiencing that divine inner light of awareness.

THOUGHTS

Any event we experience leaves an impression in our memory.

I can avoid disturbing events and participate
in positive, uplifting ones.

I will act toward others as I would like them to act toward me.

EXERCISES

Imagine how your actions might change if every moment
were recorded on video for the entire world to see.

What patterns do I possess, and how does each
one influence or drive my behavior?

If a *saṁskāra* causes negativity to arise, how can I transform that *saṁskāra* into something positive?

11

PARIṆĀMA

Transformation

परिणाम

Grant me
the serenity to accept the things I cannot change;
the courage to change the things I can;
and wisdom to know the difference.
from the SERENITY PRAYER

EVERYTHING IN NATURE, including ourselves, changes from moment to moment, day to day, year to year. How well we accept and adapt to changes can affect our lives in helpful or harmful ways. Our heart and mind can change quickly on the outside, but our deeply held opinions and longstanding habits are much slower to transform.

According to yoga and modern science, all matter is made up of basic elements, such as iron, oxygen, and tin. These elements never fundamentally change. Yet they take on different forms and combine into thousands of different molecules and composites. For example, gold remains gold even when it changes into a wedding ring, goes into a computer chip, or adorns a sculpture. We can always melt it down again and return to its original elemental state of gold.

Each person's field of consciousness is like the gold. It can go through many, many changes over time that, on the outside, make it seem as though people are quite dissimilar. Yet inside we all share the same inner light of awareness. The strong winds of a hurricane swirl around on the outside, while in the center, the eye is clear and still and unaffected by the storm. In the same way, our thoughts and emotions fluctuate around an inner light of awareness (*puruṣa*) that silently watches them.

Changes in our physical body affect our breath, heart, and mind, and vice versa. Improving the health of these three components of our human system contributes directly to our well-being and happiness. Yoga postures, breathing exercises, what and how we eat, day-to-day activities and interactions, as well as sitting quietly, all serve this end.

Rapid change is rarely sustainable, with the exception of change due to a trauma or a very intense and life-changing event. Real, lasting change usually happens gradually over time, often without us even being aware it is going on. Reading the news, traveling, holding different jobs, and experiencing relationships all cause changes in our being. Every interaction we experience is recorded in our heart and mind and contributes to who we are. Change is difficult to perceive while it is happening, especially when the change occurs slowly, over a long period of time. Only at the end of the series of changes, when things stop changing, can we fully understand each step that led us to the end result.

Unwanted or unexpected change can cause suffering. What do we do when our life changes in ways beyond our control or in ways we did not intend? The Serenity Prayer counsels us well in this regard. Events that cannot be undone, such as the loss of a limb or the death of a loved one, are to be accepted over time so we can move forward. Other events can be carefully navigated using keen discernment (*viveka*) in order to bring about as positive an outcome as possible.

Intentional change can be difficult and uncomfortable. The easiest way to change is to map out small steps toward a realistic goal and then commit to the process. We have the power to transform harmful thoughts, words, and actions into more positive and meaningful energies. Deliberate and conscious change can move us in a more helpful direction and gradually allow the negative past to fade away behind us.

For example, you treat your employees so poorly that it causes a high turnover rate, which not only lowers morale and creates an unhappy work environment, but also costs your company a significant amount of money. By setting an intention to empower your employees by listening to their concerns and providing strong, positive words of encouragement, you can gradually transform the unhealthy and uncomfortable workplace into an environment that people enjoy working in. When their work is valued and appreciated, productivity goes up, turnover goes down, and you as an employer feel much happier. It becomes a win-win situation.

The current state of each individual heart and mind is the result of past experiences and habitual patterns. Contemplation of these changes can reveal valuable information about how they arrived in their present state. By understanding these longstanding habitual patterns, as well as our genetic traits, we can glimpse what might have happened in our past to create them and even predict how they might play out in the future.

If we surround ourselves with positive influences, remain open minded, and continue to learn new, helpful things, then naturally the changes that occur will be positive and contribute to happiness. If, on the other hand, we acquiesce to negativity or stagnation, and think we do not have any control over our situation, we will move away from yoga and toward potential unhappiness and sorrow.

Nature (*dṛśya* or *prakṛti*) constantly changes, just as the cells in our bodies are continuously transforming themselves and being recycled into other substances. Because everything is always changing, clinging to anything is ultimately futile. The tug of change ever so gradually pulls on each object in this world, and as we tug against it, we inevitably encounter some degree of discomfort (*duḥkha*). Live in nature's ebb and flow, change and grow with it, feel the discomfort of resistance, and let it go.

THOUGHTS

Real, lasting change usually begins with discomfort
and ends with joy and respect for oneself.

I can replace obstructions to my progress with what
encourages and supports moving in a positive direction.

I will set an intention for positive changes in my
life that are conducive to the practice of yoga.

EXERCISES

Think about some aspect of yourself that you'd like to change. Create a plan to gradually transform this aspect. As you follow your plan, observe yourself each time you either behave as before or succeed in modifying your behavior. (These moments may be noticeable only if you sit quietly at the end of the day and ponder the day's events.) Over time, you may need to adjust your plan until it works and you feel positive about the results.

Recall a time in your life when change was thrust upon you, such as a job ending or an unexpected diagnosis of cancer. How did you react to this change? Consider how you might react differently the next time you experience an unexpected turn of events, in terms of staying positive and moving forward with your life instead of letting the event pull you down.

How are you different than you were ten or twenty years ago? Think about what caused these changes. Were they intentional or a natural result of your surroundings (people, places, or events in history)? If intentional, how did you influence others by your example?

PART 2

UNDERSTANDING SUFFERING

12

DUḤKHA

Suffering as Opportunity

दुःख

The dark thought, the shame, the malice,
meet them at the door laughing,
and invite them in.
Be grateful for whoever comes,
because each has been sent
as a guide from beyond.
RUMI

HOW WE CHOOSE TO VIEW anything, including something unpleasant, affects our relationship to it. *Duḥkha*, literally "bad space," in yoga primarily means discomfort or suffering within our heart-mind (*citta*). By exercising keen discernment (*viveka*) before making a decision or engaging in action, we can minimize or avoid altogether any negativity that may have resulted from choosing differently. When we do experience *duḥkha*, we can try and understand what caused it and how to prevent it from happening again.

If we anticipate suffering, we may be able to avoid it. For example, let's say your mother comes to visit you on a regular basis. Each time she stays for a week, there seems to be some unavoidable tension between her and your family. You ponder when and why this tension occurs, and realize that it is strongest on the day she arrives and the day she leaves. So the next time she comes, you pay extra attention to her on the first and last days of her visit and thereby reduce much of the uncomfortable tension.

Sometimes we know in our gut that if we follow through with an action, it will result in suffering. Yet we do it anyway when our habitual patterns override our good intentions. For example, you are a woman in her early thirties who wants children and you become romantically attached to a man who is on the fence about having kids. After many good years together, you turn forty and realize that your biological clock is running out. Your partner says he does not want children. At that point, you can choose to end the relationship and seek another man who wants children, or you can continue and accept that you would rather be with him than have children. Having to make this choice may cause a lot of regret and resentment toward your partner. It may have been better to, early on, consider only men who want to have children.

Duḥkha provides you with valuable information about yourself that would otherwise be hard to come by. In the midst of a painful experience, the heart-mind may be clouded, making it difficult to understand why the situation is happening. Afterward, we can step back and think about why it was painful to us. What did this event trigger inside of us that caused our suffering? Thus, we can learn what we are all about on the inside from *duḥkha*, and use it as a tool to reveal aspects of ourselves.

The *sūtra-s* mention suffering due to change, suffering due to what we want, and suffering due to what we are used to. Change happening too quickly or too slowly for us can cause suffering in the form of frustration or impatience. For example, you are naturally inflexible and are practicing yoga postures diligently. When you practice too hard, injury results, and you have to take a break. When your practice is too mild and you do not progress as quickly as you wanted, you may become frustrated to the point where you feel like quitting altogether and spending time on something else. Accepting the pace at which your body can change and practicing accordingly can help you avoid this form of suffering.

The inability to satisfy our desires—when we want change, but it doesn't happen—causes suffering as well. For example, we are driving a beat-up, fifteen-year-old car. Even though we really want a newer car, we will never be able to afford it. So when a friend who has a nice new car, with all the bells and whistles, take us out in it, we experience a bit of envy and frustration.

If discomfort arises when something we are used to changes beyond our control—when a change happens that we don't want—*duḥkha* is there, too. For example, you and your husband have been living in the same house for twenty years when he is transferred to a job in a foreign country. Because of the new country's vastly different cultural norms, you are forced to completely change your lifestyle and daily routines. This kind of unexpected and/or unwelcome transition can be painful.

Greed is a form of suffering that can grow stronger over time. First, we want more than we need, and then we begin taking from others when necessary. Finally, even though we are already wealthy, we stoop to deceit and corruption to get more. Another manifestation of suffering is anger, which can grow from annoyance to verbal jabs to violence. Delusion is also a type of *duḥkha*, and can range from simply thinking we know what we do not to full-on schizophrenia.

There are four stages to reducing suffering, much like the four noble truths of Buddhism. First, identify the symptoms of suffering. Second, find its cause. Third, set an intention of eliminating the cause. Last, put into practice the means of eliminating the cause. The triad of tools within *kriyā-yoga* are designed to diminish future suffering.

We can also reduce future suffering by looking closely at how our habitual patterns determine our reactions, listening to and watching people we respect and consider wise, and finally, using our own discrimination before embarking on a decision or action.

Suffering can be viewed as a difficult but necessary way that the universe reveals ourselves to us. It is important to set a deliberate intention to identify and reduce *duḥkha*, and then follow up that intention with on-the-ground action in order to move in our desired direction of mental, emotional, and spiritual growth and transformation. If we are mindful of this long-term commitment, we can avoid much suffering by using keen discernment to anticipate possible future pain, then taking action to bypass it.

THOUGHTS

Suffering offers insight into my deeply
held patterns and conditioning.

If I learn from the mistakes and misfortunes experienced by
myself and others, then I can avoid or reduce future suffering.

I strive to make conscious choices with
a discerning heart-mind.

Exercises

Think of a painful experience. What could you have done differently to avoid it, and what can you do to keep it from happening again?

What valuable lessons have you learned from your mistakes? Write down several "mistakes" and how learning from them contributed to your personal growth and happiness.

How might contemplation and discernment (*viveka*) help you better change and find the opportunity within suffering?

13

SAṀYOGA

False Identification of the Seer with the Seen

संयोग

All that is visible clings to the invisible,
the audible to the inaudible, the tangible to the intangible,
perhaps the thinkable to the unthinkable.
from NOVALIS, translated by Lama Govinda

THE SCIENCE OF YOGA AS presented by Patañjali presupposes a divine inner light of awareness (*puruṣa*) that invisibly pervades the entire manifest world (*dṛśya* or *prakṛti*). Like sugar dissolved in water, they are two distinct entities eternally joined so as to appear the same. *Saṁyoga* means mistakenly thinking that these two entities are the same. This basic blunder prevents us from connecting with our *puruṣa*.

Saṁyoga literally means "confusion." If a piece of black glass, representing the manifest world, is overlaid on a piece of clear glass, representing our inner light of awareness, our eyes see only black glass. The only way to distinguish between the two is to turn our attention inward and experience that which cannot be perceived by our external sensory organs. The concepts of time, space, and even language are qualities of the ever-changing manifest world; they do not exist in, nor can they be applied to, the unchanging conscious awareness. A clear and quiet heart-mind allows the deep insight necessary to connect with that true divine essence within us.

A practical way to view *saṁyoga* is as simply being too close to a situation to see it clearly. If there is no space for observation, we lack a proper perspective, which can cause suffering (*duḥkha*). For example, you found a spiritual guru who has initiated you into his lineage. After you practice loyally and faithfully with him for many years, the guru's reputation comes crashing down as evidence of impropriety with female devotees comes to light. If you are so loyal that you believe the guru's claims that he is innocent instead of the overwhelming evidence against him, then you remain in the delusional realm of ignorance. Your perspective is so narrow that you cannot accept the truth and what it means. But the ability to separate yourself from what you are involved in and to observe a situation or event from a distance allows you to put what you perceive in the proper perspective.

Avidyā, the shroud of ignorance covering our inner light of awareness, causes *saṁyoga* by preventing our heart-mind from seeing clearly. Thus, we superimpose the seer and the seen, empowering our ego and keeping ourselves trapped in the changing cycles of the manifest world. When the *puruṣa* and *citta* are taken as one and the same thing and identified as part of the individual's sense of "I," then the mental-emotional affliction called *asmitā* has reared its proud head. For example, if you think that you are your body, that you are your thoughts and emotions, then you are identifying yourself in an outer way, equating your "I" to a constantly changing set of objects. Once you recognize your divine inner nature as a permanent light of awareness around which all else changes, then the false superimposition of *saṁyoga* disappears.

Turning our attention inward enables us to gradually distinguish between what sees (*puruṣa*) and what is seen (*dṛśya* or *prakṛti*). When the veil of ignorance is lifted and we observe the world exactly as it is, without distortion, then *saṁyoga* ends, suffering ends, and true freedom begins.

THOUGHTS

An unbiased yet well-informed perspective is the best way to understand any situation.

I can recognize when I am too involved in a situation to perceive it clearly and fairly.

I will strive to step back and discriminate between impermanent, changing events and the eternal, inner light of awareness.

EXERCISES

Think of a situation in which you were too involved to be able to perceive it clearly. How would it have helped if you could have stepped back and gained a more objective view?

Meditate on your inner light of awareness in order to experience it as a separate, ever-present entity.

Mix some sugar in some water and watch the sugar dissolve.
Taste the invisible sweetness and think of that sweet,
invisible inner light of awareness that resides in your body.

14

VṚTTI-S

Activity in the Heart-Mind

वृत्ति

Wisdom arrives inside the circle;
affairs are left outside the gate.
ZEN MASTER HONGZHI

WHEN OUR LIVES BECOME BUSY and full, the heart-mind tries its best to keep track of the bottomless to-do list, so many decisions to be made, and new experiences to remember. *Vṛtti-s*, "turnings or cyclings," include all thoughts and emotions that spin around in our heart-mind and keep us preoccupied. One goal of yoga is to calm and quiet the heart-mind so these activities no longer distract us.

There are five *vṛtti-s*, which will each be described in separate chapters. They are *pramāṇa* (valid means of perception/evaluation), *viparyaya* (misperception), *vikalpa* (imagination), *nidrā* (sleep), and *smṛti* (memory).

Vṛtti-s are not necessarily bad. They can be harmful or not, depending on what caused them and how they influence our behavior. If they distort our perception or negatively affect our thoughts, words, or deeds, they are harmful. If they contribute to clarity and calmness, they are helpful. Otherwise they are neutral.

Harmful thoughts and emotions are caused by our deep mental-emotional triggers (*kleśa-s*), which are strengthened via negative impressions and behavioral patterns (*saṁskāra-s*). Whenever our actions result in some form of suffering or we experience something disturbing, the recorded memory will support future harmful thoughts and emotions. For example, let's say you are overly sensitive to even constructive criticism. Every time a friend wishes to make you aware that your action was inappropriate or hurtful, you become defensive and angry at him. This touchiness will not only harm your friend, who is just trying to help you, but may even cause him to stop trying to help you at all. Your triggers are effectively reinforcing themselves, dragging you down into a small-minded world of ignorance and rigidity.

Our ego can make us think that these outer, distracting activities define who we are. If we let this false identification happen, then our perceptions and actions will be influenced by the *vṛtti-s*, and we will remain stuck in the mire of delusion. It is important to understand that the core of our being is always quiet and still, and that core is what we want to identify with. The *vṛtti-s* spin like wheels, while the center of the wheel, the hub, stays still.

Helpful *vṛtti-s* arise from experiences and actions that produce positive energy. Acting with kindness or compassion, telling the truth, and generally living our life in an ethical and conscious way (by practicing the *yama-s* and *niyama-s*) create helpful and healthy thoughts and feelings. These positive *vṛtti-s* can be cultivated by means of yoga, and over time, they bring us closer to calming (*nirodha*) the heart-mind.

The positive *vṛtti-s* increase as the harmful ones decrease and the *kleśa-s* weaken (via *kriyā-yoga*). It is important to be aware of the distorting and painful nature of harmful *vṛtti-s.* Helpful *vṛtti-s* do not have the afflictive quality of the *kleṣa-s* in them. They promote a peaceful and clear heart-mind.

Meditation (*dhyāna*) quiets the heart-mind and calms the *vṛtti-s.* When we attempt to meditate or stay focused in some way, thoughts usually pop up to distract our attention. Diligent, regular, committed practice (*abhyāsa*) helps to reduce our desire for external objects (*vairāgya*) and, in doing so, diminishes the *vṛtti-s* in our consciousness. As we cultivate these two pillars of yoga (*abhyāsa* and *vairāgya*), along with keen discernment (*viveka*), the quelling of these activities (*nirodha*) and the clarification of the heart-mind (*citta-prasādana*) follow. Just plain slowing down the pace of our life can cultivate stillness and introspection.

THOUGHTS

The activity on the surface of the heart-mind
can conceal our inner light of awareness.

Practicing yoga includes doing everything I can
to cultivate a calm and stable heart-mind.

I will reduce distracting and harmful thoughts
by practicing meditation regularly, even if it
is for only a few minutes each day.

EXERCISES

Think of a time when a preconceived notion has caused you to judge someone unfairly, possibly based on a stereotype. How can you prevent this from happening again?

Sit quietly in meditation and observe how thoughts and emotions distract your attention from the point of focus.

Try and separate the detrimental thoughts and emotions from the helpful ones, and then investigate where the negative ones came from.

15

PRAMĀṆA

Correct Evaluation

प्रमाण

Lead me from untruth to truth.
Lead me from darkness to light.
Lead me from death to immortality
ŚRĪ GURU STOTRAM

PRAMĀṆA MEANS CORRECT PERCEPTION—literally to measure or gauge what is in front of us." In order to perceive an object or situation accurately and completely, a broad understanding is often necessary. Personal agendas, external labels, and preconceived notions can all interfere with *pramāṇa*. Each of us has our own unique life experience, which determines how we perceive the world.

What we are exposed to, and choose to expose ourselves to, heavily influences our opinions and beliefs. Sometimes we end up seeing and listening to news or gossip that is simply untrue or misleading. Choosing our sources of information wisely, easier now with the advent of the Internet, can lead us from untruth to truth. Since there are so many vastly different views on any single idea or event, it is imperative to seek out several opinions before settling on our own. Those who seek medical treatment know this all too well. Extend this idea to any piece of important information, especially if it will impact your future perceptions and actions.

There are three kinds of *pramāṇa*, in order of importance, all of which require *viveka* (discernment) to maximize the reliability of the information and decide if it is helpful or harmful.

1. Direct perception, or firsthand knowledge, where nothing stands between the heart-mind and the object being perceived by the senses. This is experiential knowledge, the most reliable kind of knowledge because it is based on our actual experience. Can we know what honey tastes like if someone merely describes it to us in words?

2. Inference, or secondhand knowledge. The mind is involved here, inferring information based on what is perceived. For example, when you see smoke, the mind infers there is a fire, even though you cannot see the fire. If what you see is not smoke, but something else not caused by a fire, your inference that there is a fire is incorrect, because it was based on a misperception (*viparyaya*).

3. Reliable testimony, or second- or thirdhand knowledge often gleaned from reading a book or hearing from another person. Traditionally this knowledge comes from texts written by people who are considered reliable, who have had direct experience of their own. This kind of perception requires our own verification from direct experience. Testimony informs and reinforces our own direct perception.

Learning involves all of these types of perception. Sometimes we obtain information from a teacher or books, then infer and extrapolate, and wait to see if the information holds up to direct experience. Or we may witness something first, which is then reinforced by what we read or hear from others. Inference is based on what we think we know, which comes from direct perception or testimony. In the end, we must judge something to be correct based on what we know. A clear heart-mind is able to observe events accurately, as they are, and remember them truthfully.

Correct perception can be either helpful or harmful. A helpful or neutral *pramāṇa* is simply when we perceive something accurately and it does not disturb our heart-mind. A helpful *pramāṇa* could be witnessing an act of unconditional loving-kindness, such as a person helping a complete stranger get up after taking a fall.

A harmful *pramāṇa* is when we correctly observe something that disturbs the heart-mind. For example, watching a violent movie may cause impressions in our heart-mind that will adversely affect our future actions. If we witness an event that we simply cannot process because it is so foreign to us, our heart-mind does not know how to digest it, so it becomes improperly recorded in memory. It is simply not part of our reality. This undigested material has the potential to cause confusion, just as undigested food can cause physical disease.

Be careful what you ask for. The universe has a way of listening to our thoughts and providing what is necessary to move in their direction. Before setting an intention or praying for something to happen, sit quietly and contemplate the possible consequences, both positive and negative. If our heart-mind is imbued with clarity, discernment, and compassion, we will see objects and events as they are and funnel that truth into our prayers and intentions. True thoughts, honest communication, and right action naturally follow, leading to positive, accurate memories that will then support these qualities in our heart-mind in a recurring cycle that develops and refines our field of consciousness.

THOUGHTS

The highest and most reliable form of
knowledge is direct, firsthand perception.

With a clear an open heart-mind, I can
register external events accurately.

I will carefully choose my secondary sources of
information, including teachers, books, and news.

EXERCISES

Pick an important issue and ask three people
that you respect for their opinions on it.

For your next big decision, collect opinions about
it from close friends or family members, as well
as other sources, if appropriate. See how this
extra knowledge affects your final decision.

Make a list of qualities that may indicate when a news
source is biased or skewed. Keep your eyes and ears open
for these qualities when you are exposed to the media.

16

VIPARYAYA

Misperception

विपर्यय

We do not see things as they are.
We see them as we are.
THE TALMUD

VIPARYAYA, PERCEIVING SOMETHING INCORRECTLY, is the opposite of *pramāṇa* (correct perception). Misperception can be due to lack of information, false assumptions, or our own distorted process of perceiving. This *vṛtti* is caused by a lack of knowledge or understanding (*avidyā*) and is to be removed by clarifying our heart-mind (*citta-prasādana*).

Sometimes we think we understand something, but we do not yet have enough information for a full picture. An example is the blessing in disguise. A man falls off a horse and breaks his leg. This injury seems unfortunate until a war breaks out, and all the men in the town are called upon to fight, except the man who broke his leg. His life may now be spared because the injury was a blessing in the end. Accepting events as they occur and moving forward with a positive and hopeful attitude enables us to bypass unnecessary suffering and anxiety.

The harmful form of *viparyaya* is delusion, when perception and reality do not match. If we are used to looking at things in a certain way and our expectations are not met, then our misperception is due to past conditioning (*saṁskāra-s*), and we suffer. Our ego, responsible for maintaining our reputation, or "saving face," may prevent us from admitting we are wrong. This unbending attitude will alienate us from the truth and lead to actions based on incorrect information.

When we make assumptions based on incomplete knowledge, thinking we are right when we are actually wrong, then *viparyaya* is present. For example, in the dark you see on the ground something long, skinny, and twisted, and you think it is a snake. When daylight appears, you see that the object is clearly just a rope. Your original perception of the object as a snake is *viparyaya*. Your corrected perception—it is a rope—is *pramāṇa*.

Judgments based on misperception can be quite wrong and unfair. Limited interaction with certain groups of people who may share a common racial background can lead to stereotyping and racism. If we, after one or two negative experiences with members of a certain race, then expect everyone who fits that racial profile to be like those who were involved in our negative experiences, then we have moved away from yoga and toward prejudice and racism.

Just because something or someone is foreign to us and we have a limited understanding of them is no reason to make broad judgments. If we read a single article about someone who fell sick after ingesting an herb, is it fair to blame and avoid the entire science of herbalism? It would be wiser to seek out professional herbalists and ask them why the person became ill.

A helpful form of *viparyaya* is its transformation into correct perception (*pramāṇa*) by admitting we are wrong, asking questions to verify our perception, and/or adjusting our knowledge to fit reality. Learning from our mistakes and listening to different perspectives helps to reduce *viparyaya* and increase *pramāṇa.*

By clarifying our heart-mind (*citta-prasādana*) and refining our sensory organs to the point where they are keen, alert, and fully under our control, we can reduce the likelihood of false perception and increase our ability to see things as they actually are. Open-mindedness and the capacity to learn from and move through our life experiences will lead to fewer unfair misperceptions and more understanding of the people and events around us.

THOUGHTS

What I perceive is not always the truth.

I can adjust my opinions and behavior as I encounter new and better information.

I will strive to see things as they are at all times and not jump to unfair conclusions..

EXERCISES

Ask a friend to tell you when you are wrong. When your friend does, notice what comes up in you.

Choose one political event in the news and collect opinions about it from several different news channels or political commentators. Try and discern what makes sense and what is accurate, keeping in mind the background of each information source. How can you tell if someone is motivated by money or fame as opposed to being interested in the greater good?

Have another person talk about his or her background and notice what presumptions you make. Are your presumptions all accurate? Are they fair?

17

VIKALPA

Imagination

विकल्प

Sit in reverie and watch the changing color of the waves
that break upon the idle seashore of the mind.
HENRY WADSWORTH LONGFELLOW from *The Spanish Student*

VIKALPA IS AN IDEA OR abstraction that has no basis in reality. It comes from a concept in the heart-mind that does not actually exist. Real knowledge is supported by fact and is antagonistic to *vikalpa*. Yet *vikalpa* serves the purpose of creating abstract thoughts, which may eventually manifest in a practical way (like mathematics) or lead to a higher level of understanding beyond our limited intellect.

Some words like *infinite* or *possible* have no real objects and could be construed as *vikalpa*. A phrase like "pie in the sky" really does mean something as an idiom and, therefore, will create activity in the heart-mind. Some ideas used in conversation carry a variety of interpretations, depending on the background of the speaker. Even the concept of a higher power or divinity, such as *puruṣa*, is a *vikalpa*, albeit a nonharmful one.

Daydreams can be harmful if they distract our attention from something important. For example, driving a car while daydreaming may cause an accident. Daydreaming in a classroom during an important lecture may cause us to miss key points. Fantasies also have the potential to be detrimental. If our heart-mind is preoccupied with a fantasy about becoming rich based on a shaky get-rich-quick scheme, our attention has turned outward, into the world of possessions and success. If we make decisions based on this unrealistic fantasy, we are likely to suffer. In this way, *vikalpa* can contribute to misperception (*viparyaya*) and delusion. Any ideas or imaginings that occur in our *citta* should not pull us away from our chosen focus and practice of yoga.

Daydreams can be helpful if they are uplifting. Thinking of yourself winning a race or imagining yourself being flexible enough to do a full split are examples of uplifting daydreams. Visualizing yourself in a healthy and loving relationship will have a positive impact on your psyche and may energetically help materialize that wish.

Additionally, ideas that seem crazy or impossible or totally impractical when they occur can lead to significant discoveries and useful inventions. High-level abstract thinking, such as the kind involved in theoretical mathematics or musical composition, challenges the brain and cultivates forward thinking and creativity. A teacher or parent can inspire a student or child to try out ideas and see if they can become reality. Imaginative play can stimulate a child's brain in a very healthy way. Keeping our heart and mind open to unforeseen possibilities helps us grow, progress, and improve.

If the *vikalpa* is linked to realistic possibilities, it can be helpful. For example, let's say you do not like your current job, but stay in it for the money or prestige. You feel there is no other possibility. But if you spend time imagining what you really want to do, you may be able to come up with a way to actualize your desire. Maybe you can take classes at a local college and get another degree that will help you move in that new direction. Many people have gone through yoga teachers' training while working, then quit their job to pursue teaching yoga full time, for example.

Believing in concepts like *puruṣa*, our pure inner light of awareness, can make us feel less attached to the outer world. The experience of that divine presence, often found via meditation, can actually affect our outer behavior in a positive way.

Imagination that diverts our attention and causes present or future suffering is to be avoided. Ruminations and constructive ideas that support or enhance our yoga practice and our lives, or the lives of others, are to be encouraged. As long as our hearts and minds are focused on cultivating inner awareness and improving outer behavior, positive imaginings can help. May we keep our hearts and minds open to fresh and bright possibilities and not allow others to stifle our ideas.

THOUGHTS

Imagination and fantasy can bring me joy as well as suffering.

I choose to use my imagination for creative
thinking and self-reflection.

I will make important decisions with a heart-mind
grounded in reality yet inspired by possibilities.

Exercises

The next time you notice yourself daydreaming in a way that may be detrimental to your heart-mind, try and shift your attention to something positive and/or productive.

Think of ways in which imagination has cut you off from reality, in both helpful and harmful ways.

Examine some of your hopes and dreams. How possible are they? What steps can you take to eventually reach them?

18

NIDRĀ

Sleep

निद्रा

Whatever is the night of all beings,
in that the yogī is awake.
Whatever all beings are awake in,
that is the night for the yogī who sees.
BHAGAVAD GĪTĀ 2.69

WE SPEND ABOUT ONE-THIRD OF our life sleeping for the purpose of resting our body and mind. Too much or too little sleep can cause sloth or nervousness, respectively, and both are obstacles (*antarāya-s*) to yoga. Though sleep and meditation may appear the same on the outside, deep, dreamless sleep is heavy and unconscious, while deliberately meditating inwardly is alert and conscious.

There are four sleep states: wakefulness, dream sleep, deep (dreamless) sleep, and beyond. Wakefulness, when our attention is projected outward, is considered a state of sleep since true awakening happens only when our attention is focused inward. The Bhagavad Gītā verse above implies that whatever a living being does not see (the inner light of awareness), the yogin can, and whatever a living being does see (sensory perceptions), the yogin does not (is not distracted by those). Here, a yogin is one who practices *saṁyama* (turning inward).

In dream sleep, lots of activity is taking place in our heart-mind, based upon our thoughts and emotions earlier that day and upon our previous memories. When harmful *vṛtti-s* occur during this unconscious sleep state, they can tarnish the psyche and affect our behavior in the future. Dream sleep is similar to, yet different from the initial stages of turning inward (*saṁyama*). Training our heart-mind to focus on a single point is done consciously and deliberately, even as those pesky *vṛtti-s* do their best to distract our attention. Dream sleep also involves the noise of thoughts and feelings dancing around in our heads, yet it is completely unconscious.

Deep sleep is similar to, yet different from *samādhi*, the final limb of yoga. Like *samādhi*, deep sleep is restful to the body and calming to the heart-mind. Yet deep sleep is unconscious and involuntary, whereas *samādhi* is conscious and voluntary. In deep sleep, the *citta* is enveloped by darkness (*tamas*), and the seer within witnesses blackness. In *samādhi*, the *citta* is clear and filled with light (*sattva*), which allows us to experience our pure inner light of awareness.

The fourth sleep state is not even a sleep state per se; it is beyond sleep. The heart and mind are utterly and completely still. We are not even aware that full awareness is occurring.

Nidrā can also mean sleepiness, and in the *sūtra-s* it is indeed described as heavy and dulling (*tamas*). Sleepiness is helpful if we are naturally tired and then get the rest that our body and mind require. However, if you are at a meeting where you are supposed to be attentive, and you nod off in the middle and miss some important information, then sleepiness is not good for you. In the same way, if you sit to meditate and end up falling asleep, then you cannot go as deeply inward as if you were completely alert.

Consciously remembering and focusing on the calmness we experience during sleep can clarify the heart-mind and effect that state in it. Exposing ourselves to happy and easy-to-digest impressions will reduce nightmares and promote pleasant dreams, which, in turn, will exert a positive influence on our everyday thoughts and emotions.

THOUGHTS

Deep, dreamless sleep is restful yet unconscious.
Meditation is restful and conscious.

I can protect and cherish the time I set
aside for deep, restful sleep.

I will meditate when I am alert and awake,
not when I am tired and sleepy.

EXERCISES

During the day, take a moment to focus on the inner light of awareness instead of all the sights, sounds, and other sensations of the outside world. Keep reminding yourself that the pure, radiant, inner world is what connects us all.

Think of ways you can prevent yourself from falling asleep during meditation, like choosing a better time of day to meditate or making sure you are not tired beforehand.

Compare how you feel when you wake up from sleep to how you feel after a long session of meditation. Write down what you remember about your sleep versus your meditation.

19

SMṚTI

Memory

स्मृति

It's surprising how much of memory is built
around things unnoticed at the time.
BARBARA KINGSOLVER

EVERY TIME WE ACT OR think or speak, we draw from our memory. Therefore, what we remember directly affects our behavior and the way we perceive the outside world. If we are to act in a kinder and gentler manner, then we must be careful and vigilant with what we expose ourselves to.

Like all *vṛtti-s*, memories can be helpful, harmful, or neutral. An uplifting movie can become a helpful memory if it is positive and contributes to our happiness. A helpful and constructive form of *smṛti* could be memorizing something useful or repeating a mantra over and over again until it penetrates into the depth memory. On the other hand, watching a film with violence or horror may cause nightmares or violent imitative actions, creating detrimental memories that can lead to future suffering. A neutral form of memory might be the phantom-limb phenomenon. When individuals lose an arm or leg, often their mind thinks it is still there, and they can actually feel sensations from their nonexistent hand or foot.

Everything we experience is recorded in our memory. A strong impression in our memory may last much longer than we expect. Memories of loved ones who died long ago, of songs we have heard, of joy we have experienced, are all retained in our *smṛti.* There are times when we consciously do something to keep a memory alive, such as visiting a loved one's gravesite or reviewing material so it stays fresh in our mind.

Memory can influence *saṁskāra-s,* and vice versa. When we witness or participate in an event that is very intense or repeated many times, the memory of that event is stronger, stores deeper in our *citta,* and can therefore contribute to habitual tendencies (*saṁskāra-s*). When these stored patterns of behavior are negative or detrimental, they become psycho-emotional baggage that we carry with us all the time, and they influence our actions and reactions. Deep in our memory, negative *saṁskāra-s* strengthen the *kleṣa-s,* while positive, helpful *saṁskāra-s* weaken them. Inaccurate or harmful memories manifest as afflicted thoughts and emotions (*kliṣṭa-vṛtti-s*) that distort our perceptions and negatively affect our actions.

The clarity of our heart-mind determines how accurately an experience is stored in our memory. Whatever we *think* we saw or heard is what gets stored in our memory. Correct perception (*pramāṇa*) means the stored memories are truthful, while misperception (*viparyaya*) leads to untruthful memories. Clarification and purification of our heart-mind (*citta-prasādana*) is essential for seeing the world as it actually is.

The process of yoga includes the gradual replacement of harmful or negative memories with helpful or positive ones. Whatever receives attention will strengthen, and whatever we pay no attention to will weaken. As we pay less attention to detrimental habits and give more attention to those that are beneficial, eventually the former are superseded by the latter. This process reprograms the heart-mind and moves us toward happiness and optimism.

If we are brought up to think certain things are true or right, then we will perceive and act based upon those premises. We are products of our experiences and highly impressionable at a young age. For example, let's say a person is raised in a "might makes right" environment, where all issues are ultimately resolved through fighting. As an adult, this person will see the world in much the same way as wild animals do, through the narrow lens of "survival of the fittest." On the other hand, someone brought up with love and trust will view their environment with much less fear believing in cooperation rather than competition.

The clarity of our heart-mind also affects our communication and understanding. For example, a little boy's mother dies, and his father remarries a woman who is not loving toward him. As an adult, the boy marries a woman who truly loves him. But one day, he does something that she does not like, and she lets him know. Because of his past conditioning, he interprets what she says to mean that she does not love him. His wife said one thing, but he heard another, thereby creating a negative impression in his heart and mind. Mirroring is an excellent way to prevent such miscommunication from happening. If there is any potential for misunderstanding, repeating back what the person said enables us to confirm what we heard and, thus, avoid further problems. Mirroring will strengthen instead of weaken a relationship.

Memory is necessary for reminding the heart-mind to stay on its point of focus. The deeper purpose of *smṛti* is to remember our true nature. When the *smṛti* is completely purified, then we can experience our pure inner light of awareness.

THOUGHTS

Clear, accurate perceptions can replace
past, inaccurate impressions.

What I remember will create an impression
that can affect my behavior.

I will remember to engage in that which is
conducive to the practice of yoga.

EXERCISES

Choose something easy that you want to learn, like a song or *sūtra*, and repeat it so many times that it becomes part of you.

The next time you notice a potential misunderstanding about to happen between you and someone else, clarify what the other person said up front to make sure that you heard it correctly.

Think of activities you do that may be detrimental to your spiritual growth. Can you modify them or replace them with more positive and inwardly satisfying activities?

20

ANTARĀYA-S

Obstacles That Distract

अन्तराय

Opportunities to find deeper powers within ourselves come when life seems most challenging.
JOSEPH CAMPBELL

WHEN WE TAKE THE TIME to sit quietly and turn our attention inward, it is important that our body is comfortable, our breath flows freely, and our heart-mind is alert. *Antarāya-s* are obstacles that divert our attention from the point of focus. All nine obstacles are disruptions to the heart-mind field of consciousness (*citta*) and can be debilitating to a practice, because distracting thoughts and emotions (*vṛtti-s*) arise when *antarāya-s* are present. These nine obstacles are disease, apathy, self-doubt, carelessness, fatigue, sexual preoccupation, erroneous views, ungroundedness, and regression.

1. Disease or illness can be a major distraction and may be extremely difficult to remove. This is the only obstacle that does not necessarily come from a *kleśa*. It is the most external of the distractions, involves the physical body, and can

originate outside the body. Maintaining a quiet, focused heart-mind while sniffling, sneezing, or feeling physical pain after surgery is quite a challenge. Yet a fully focused heart-mind can actually cut off the pain signals to the brain.

2. Disease can easily lead to the second obstacle, apathy, or an attitude of not caring about anything. When we become ill with a headache, sore throat, or fever, our alertness and zest are replaced by a groggy disinterest in everyday activities. Knowing the discomfort is temporary can help us patiently allow the sickness to run its course. A more serious disease or injury can extend our apathetic state for much longer. Whatever the cause, this dullness prevents us from converting thoughts into actions. Stimulation of our heart-mind by means of vigorous *āsana*, active *prāṇāyāma* practice, or some other stimulating exercise can get us out of this state.

3. Apathy can give rise to self-doubt, or lack of confidence, which is particularly arresting since it can cause us to stop our practice for a while. Like fire, self-doubt can consume everything in its path and thereby affect every area of our lives. With it comes the inability to decide between two things. This kind of paralysis can be even worse than making a bad decision because we are stuck in a state of limbo. Faith in ourselves is necessary to overcome this obstacle.

4. Self-doubt can produce a state of not thinking clearly and an inability to focus our attention. If we act carelessly, without paying proper attention, we will likely cause ourselves and others potentially disastrous pain and suffering, with unknown future consequences. This obstacle is similar to being in a drunken stupor.

5. Carelessness and inattentiveness scatter the heart-mind and can lead to fatigue. When the body or mind is too exhausted to practice, it is easy to slouch on the couch or go to sleep. If we can muster the energy to sit quietly for just a few minutes, that tiny investment will enable us to maintain the helpful habit of daily practice.

6. Another obstacle to practice is sensory and sexual temptation and preoccupation, literally the inability to stay away from sensual attractions. This powerful energy can send our attention in an unhealthy and potentially obsessive direction. Sexual and sensual indulgence, often driven by the ego's quest for gratification, can be difficult to control. Decreasing our involvement with external things (*vairāgya*) and investing our time and energy in turning our attention inward will cause our interest in these temptations to diminish.

7. Erroneous or distorted views of the world are similar to misperception (*viparyaya*). Delusion, not seeing reality as it is, clouds and twists sensory information coming into the heart-mind and stores it inaccurately in memory, leading to biased future thoughts and actions. Someone with a rigid or extreme philosophical stance, such as being too righteous, literal, or fundamentalist, is prone to error since there are many paths to the same spiritual goal. The practice of yoga requires the ability to let go of our opinions and consider other viewpoints as valid.

8. The inability to remain grounded at one level of development prevents us from progressing further. For all but a few rare beings, yoga, as a process, occurs in stages. If we try and move on without being firmly grounded in the previous stages, we cannot progress fully. We are, in a sense, off balance, teetering

between moving forward or backward. For example, you try to meditate without having your breath (*prāṇa*) under control. Since your breath directly affects your nervous system and mind, there is no way to become internally quiet, which is necessary for you to move through the stages of turning inward (*saṁyama*).

9. Instability or regression is when we have progressed, but we cannot maintain that level of focus and fall back into a previous stage. Naturally, there will be times of upward progress and growth, and plateau times when we feel like nothing is moving. During these times of apparent stagnation, patience and perseverance are crucial. The final stage (*samādhi*) of turning inward is difficult to maintain, yet with diligent practice, its duration will gradually lengthen.

These obstacles have symptoms or effects associated with them: pain (physical or mental), negativity/dejection, trembling, and disturbed breathing. One may lead to another, in the order mentioned. Inner suffering negatively affects the heart-mind, leading to upset or frustration, which can cause nervousness and twitching of the limbs, which affect inhalation and exhalation patterns.

The *antarāya-s* are major distractions that get in the way of our inward-focused attention. According to the *sūtra-s*, diligent practice (*abhyāsa*) can prevent the obstacles from distracting our attention. Repeating the *praṇara*, which in India is most commonly the *Om* mantra, can make them go away completely by dissolving them in the original sound of the universe.

THOUGHTS

My ability to remain relaxed and focused is hindered when my body is uncomfortable or my heart-mind is not alert.

Through self-observation (*svādhyāya*), I can identify hindrances to my practice, then take steps to reduce and eliminate them.

I will develop a healthy body and calm heart-mind by practicing regularly and chanting *Om*.

EXERCISES

Choose obstacles that distract your practice and write down ways of eliminating them.

Sit quietly and chant *Om* and notice how it can take your mind off of some obstacles.

The next time you sit for meditation, notice if your body is uncomfortable or restless sitting on the floor. Then try meditating while sitting on a chair, and see if that helps reduce some obstacles or their accompanying symptoms.

21

KLEŚA-S

Mental-Emotional Afflictions

क्लेश

Seeds of unhappiness,
sources of fear,
cause conflict and strife.
Roast them with the flame of awareness
and clearly hear,
the inner essence of life.

NICOLAI BACHMAN

EMOTIONS OR INSTINCTS THAT ARISE when our buttons are pushed, causing a negative reaction instead of a positive action, are called *kleśa-s*. They are buried deep inside our being, waiting to surface at the opportune moment.

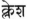

There are five *kleśa-s*, each described in detail in its own chapter. The first and most important, lack of awareness (*avidyā*), results from the other four, and they, in turn, can exist only if *avidyā* is present. *Avidyā* is the shroud of ignorance, a simple lack of knowledge that prevents us from understanding something. It is the sound chamber in which the *kleśa-s* are heard. The remaining afflictions are *asmitā* (egotism, feeling more or less than you really are), *rāga* (desire for previously experienced pleasure), *dveṣa* (aversion to previously experienced pain), and *abhiniveśa* (fear of death; the will to live, instinct to survive). Each of these, like a virus, waits inside the heart-mind for an event to trigger it. When that happens, it awakens and affects our thoughts, words, and deeds in a harmful and negative way.

All *kleśa-s* are fear based. *Avidyā* is the fear borne of ignorance. *Asmitā* is the fear the ego has of losing decision-making power or things it has become attached to. *Rāga* erupts when we are afraid we will not experience a certain pleasure again, while *dveṣa* manifests from being afraid we will endure a painful event again. *Abhiniveśa* is the deepest fear of death.

The *kleśa-s* are arguably the most challenging aspects of ourselves to confront, yet weakening and eventually removing them can be the most liberating part of our yoga practice. *Kleśa-s* cause us to suffer by producing negative thoughts and emotions (*kliṣṭa-vṛtti-s*) in our heart-mind. Yoga describes three practices, collectively known as *kriyā-yoga*, that can weaken these afflictions over time: practice causing positive change (*tapas*), self-observation (*svādhyāya*), and humility with faith (*īśvara-praṇidhāna*). These practices have the power to fundamentally change our behavioral patterns and cripple these powerful afflictions.

Kleśa-s become stronger or weaker as our behavioral patterns play out. In any situation, especially interpersonal relations, we have the capability to act consciously or react unconsciously. Every action we perform creates a subtle impression that is recorded in our memory. Performing an action over and over, or experiencing a very strong impression from an event (like a trauma), creates a memory strong enough to influence future actions. The stronger the impression, the more it can affect our action or reaction. Over time, these memories lead us to form habitual patterns strong enough to overpower our conscious mind's intention to act differently. Our mental-emotional baggage can then drive our actions, often resulting in a reaction that further reinforces the unhealthy pattern of behavior, and thus, perpetuates our suffering.

In order to actually eliminate these inner afflictions, we must understand where they came from and how they were produced (*pratiprasava*). Our current mental-emotional configuration is due to our past-life experiences. We are the sum total of what we have gone through. Tracing a negative habitual behavior back to its original cause is like finding the cause of a disease. Once that has been discovered, action can be taken to remove it.

Once the *kleśa* is rendered inert, it is unable to activate, in the same way that the volume control of an audio device becomes useless when the device is powered off. Then any related behavioral patterns will be unable to affect future actions, and no new harmful *vṛtti-s* related to that particular *kleśa* are created. Harmful thoughts and emotions (*kliṣṭa-vṛtti-s*) are like outer manifestations of the *kleśa-s*, and can be reduced by meditation (*dhyāna*).

When we weaken and nullify the *kleśa-s* using *kriyā-yoga*, then eliminate them with *pratiprasava*, they are no longer able to sprout and cause unconscious reactions. When our baggage no longer drives our actions, and our *citta* is clear, then our attention can move on toward permanent freedom (*kaivalya*).

Thoughts

Ignorance, egotism, attachment to past pleasure or pain, and the fear of death all create suffering.

I want to know why I react negatively, then take steps to lessen my reactions.

I will practice *kriyā-yoga* in order to resolve my afflictions and cultivate true inner happiness.

Exercises

Observe a typical reaction of yours, and explore when it began and why.

Write down all the ways one harmful behavioral pattern is detrimental to your life.

Why might you be afraid to dig up a deep, longstanding issue that you know needs to be worked out?

22

AVIDYĀ

Lack of Awareness

अविद्या

In darkness unawakened, they make foolishness cover their wisdom and overflow. One remembrance of illumination can break through and leap out of the dust.

ZEN MASTER HONGZHI

AVIDYĀ CAN BE A SIMPLE lack of understanding, being "in the dark" about something. It is a dark veil that cloaks our *citta*, causing us to act out of blind ignorance. *Vidyā* is the inner light of knowledge. As darkness is simply a lack of light, so *avidyā* is a lack of *vidyā* or awareness. By increasing awareness, ignorance decreases. The word *guru* means that which lightens (*ru*) the darkness (*gu*) of *avidyā* by shedding the light of knowledge on our consciousness. *Avidyā* can be eliminated by the light of knowledge, in the form of accurate information based on correct perception (*pramāṇa*) and directly experiencing our inner light of awareness (*puruṣa*).

According to yoga, the primary evil is simply a lack of knowledge or awareness (*vidyā*)—*avidyā*. When our field of consciousness becomes muddled by perceptions and actions that are harmful to ourselves or to those around us, then our divine inner light of awareness cannot shine out into the world.

Let's say our field of awareness is a window of glass. As our heart-mind accumulates the dust and dirt of worldly experience, forming rigid opinions and causing harmful thoughts and actions, the glass gradually becomes darker and darker. The dirt becomes a filter through which we see the world less and less accurately, less and less truthfully. Eventually, only a tiny fraction of our inner light can shine out through the window of awareness to illuminate our perceptions and actions. This contraction causes our field of awareness to become muddled, resulting in perceptions and actions based on fear and closed-mindedness. We now act not from knowledge, but from being "in the dark."

Avidyā is the very first *kleśa*, and, as such, carries the most importance. The other four *kleśa-s* exist in the field of *avidyā*—they need it to exist. *Avidyā* is like fertile soil in which the seeds of the other *kleśa-s* can grow and thrive. As ignorance breeds fear, so *avidyā* feeds egotism (*asmitā-kleśa*) and the other three *kleśa-s*. *Avidyā* is truly the root cause of unhappiness and discontent.

Too much commotion and busyness in the heart-mind distracts our attention and causes us to neglect the pure light of awareness that rests inside our heart-mind. Clearing the cloud of *avidyā*, which causes us to think the changeable world around us is no different than our inner light of awareness, ends suffering (*duḥkha*) and leads to the cascade of events that brings permanent freedom (*kaivalya*). *Avidyā* can be cleared away by diligent practice (*abhyāsa*) and keen discernment (*viveka*), which lead to a state of noninvolvement (*vairāgya*). A sincere effort to purify the body, breath, and heart-mind will gradually clear out impurities. As the impurities clear, our knowledge and awareness open up, illuminating the heart-mind. As darkness cannot exist in the presence of light, so ignorance disappears in the presence of knowledge.

Being open-minded contributes to learning the truth and clearing the film of *avidyā* off the lens of our *citta*. Working to weaken the other mental-emotional afflictions will gradually wipe away the grime of ignorance and allow our inner light of awareness to shine forth into the world, for the benefit of everyone around us.

THOUGHTS

The inability to perceive clearly and act consciously causes pain and suffering.

As I purify my body and heart-mind, I experience glimpses of my divine inner light.

I will vigilantly strive to weaken and neutralize the latent afflictions responsible for my suffering.

EXERCISES

Think of a situation in which your perception was clouded by your preconceived notions. To prevent this from happening again, what can you learn from that situation?

The next time you are in a restaurant where you can smell the food being prepared in the kitchen, try and isolate the smell of a single food on a single plate. Imagine the smells are the *vṛtti-s* and the single food is what you are trying to smell accurately. Removing *avidyā* is like eliminating all those smells except for that of the single food you are trying to focus on.

Picture yourself walking into a dark room, and all of a sudden, someone appears and scares you. If you had known ahead of time that the person was there, how might your reaction have been different? How much less would your level of fear be? The more you are aware of, the weaker *avidyā* is.

23

ASMITĀ

Distorted Sense of Self

अस्मिता

If you compare yourself to others, you may become
vain or bitter, for always there will be greater
and lesser persons than yourself.
MAX EHRMANN, from *Desiderata*

ASMITĀ, MEANING "I AM-NESS," is having a distorted image of ourselves that does not match reality. It is either egotism or insecurity, both of which are forms of delusion because they do not represent the truth—that we are no better or worse than anyone else. *Asmitā* is a mental-emotional affliction because it makes us think that we are our body, we are our mind, and therefore, we are our thoughts and emotions (*vṛtti-s*). It causes us to believe that our being is limited by things like our name, occupation, likes and dislikes. Yoga teaches that our exterior shell, called the body, houses a pure inner light of awareness that is our true, permanent nature. We are this inner light, not that outer form.

Some people believe they are better than others because of their accomplishments or status. The ego loves to win, and attention is its nectar. Fame and power naturally come to those who excel in certain fields. Often this fame and power can lead to conceit, pompousness, and self-centered actions. For example, a champion athlete brags after winning. A corporate executive treats her employees with derision. A wealthy person looks condescendingly at a janitor. This egotism contains an element of fear—the fear of eventually losing one's elevated position and power, which, with time, is inevitable. Few people enjoy the company of one who is arrogant or a bragger, while it is always refreshing to be around a leader or champion who is humble amid all his accolades.

Power can corrupt. The ego likes to feel powerful and in control, so it welcomes this energy. Top-down chains of command, such as corporate ladders and religious or military hierarchies, are natural and necessary for a group of people to function effectively as a team. Yet all too often, the people at the top abuse the power they've acquired because they no longer care about the "little guys" on the bottom. Once we begin to think we have power over or are in any way better than other people, the heart-mind moves away from yoga and deteriorates toward *avidyā*.

When we feel insecure and think we are less than we actually are, self-doubt rears its demoralizing head. For example, you are new to yoga and decide to attend a *yoga-āsana* class. On the mat next to you is a very advanced student. You are in pain; she is flowing like honey. Even after many weeks, it seems you will never catch up to her. Comparing yourself to others in this way can both inflate or deflate the ego, thereby engaging the *asmitā-kleśa*.

An insecure ego is terrified of relinquishing control. When it is threatened, *asmitā* arises to defend it. The ego will go to any length in order to save face and avoid feeling embarrassed in any way, including risking life itself. Sometimes we may want others to think we know more than we do and, thus, to feel a bit more powerful. This combination of outer confidence with inner ignorance and insecurity is a form of delusion and deceit, and it can lead to serious consequences in both personal and business activities. For example, a quiet high-school student is mocked relentlessly by bullies. He feels powerless and utterly humiliated. One day at school, he guns down the bullies before killing himself. His ego was able to reassert its control one last time, if only for a few moments, and would rather die powerful than live with the consequences.

An inflated ego can actually limit us. The narrow-minded view of a superiority complex closes us off from our most powerful potential—the realizations that those around us are reflections of ourselves and that treating others with kindness and respect will open doors of opportunity that would otherwise have remained closed.

A healthy ego feels content and does not feel threatened by change. Sometimes a group of people feel happy and secure because of their common way of life and belief system. When someone comes along who does not quite fit into that mold, acting differently than everyone is used to, the status quo is threatened. An ego that is rigid may be threatened by a nonconformist, even if what that individual does is actually good for the community.

When we realize that the inner heart-mind is distinct from, yet close to, the inner light of awareness, and that we are better off when the ego takes orders from the inner heart-mind, then *asmitā* will not cause us suffering. Our actions will be governed by our higher, inner intelligence, instead of the ego, whose agenda is to make us think that we are the body and our personality as defined by our thoughts and emotions (*vṛtti-s*).

Through practicing *kriyā-yoga, asmitā-kleṣa* can be weakened. To prevent pompousness, for example, we can first apply the tool of self-observation (*svādhyāya*) by noticing when we receive extra attention, then implement positive change (*tapas*) by consciously reminding ourselves that we are no better than anyone else, and finally transferring that attention to another entity (*īśvara-praṇidhāna*) by giving credit for the attention to our teachers. To prevent insecurity, we can first reflect on why we feel insecure, then make an effort to transform that feeling into something positive, and, finally, have faith that deep in the center of our impermanent, changing body glows the eternal light of awareness.

It is important to have a healthy ego in order to function in society. A weakened *asmitā* means that most of the time we neither think of ourselves as better than others nor see ourselves as less than others, and we welcome suggestions for self-improvement, even if they are difficult to hear. We are no longer embarrassed by verbal criticism and do not need to save face because our inner sense of self can withstand what it knows to be only external perceptions. As the saying goes, "Sticks and stones may break my bones, but names will never hurt me." If we let what is harmful to us pass through, and register only what is helpful to us, we will not become offended when verbal abuse comes our way.

Whatever we identify with reveals our individual nature to a certain extent. Our physical body and personality are nothing more or less than our genetic nature overlaid with our life experiences. According to yoga, deep inside each person is the same divine light of awareness that never changes and that watches the world through our clear or foggy heart and mind.

As *asmitā* weakens, we will realize that, in fact, we are better off treating others as we would like to be treated and that we are no more or less important than anybody else. Once we allow ourselves to listen to our inner, divine voice, then our ego becomes a servant instead of the master, and *asmitā-kleśa* is destroyed. We can truly embody the phrase *namaste*, which means, "I bow to and acknowledge the pure inner light of awareness within you."

THOUGHTS

Who am I really? Am I limited by the facade of external things such as my name, occupation, reputation, and preferences?

I am no more or less important than anyone else.

I will not be controlled or confined by an overinflated or underinflated sense of myself.

EXERCISES

The next time you are in a class and feel too embarrassed to ask a question, ask it anyway and then reflect on how you feel afterward.

The next time you feel peer pressure to attend an event that you really are not interested in, step back and see if you can muster the strength to say no.

Think of situations in which you perceive yourself as better than those around you. See if there is something you can learn from each and every person in that situation.

24

RĀGA

Clinging to Past Pleasure

राग

Wherever you will be attached, there you will go.
KIRPAL SINGH

WHEN WE HAVE AN EXPERIENCE that is pleasurable, it is natural to desire it again. An attachment is formed. If the desire cannot be fulfilled, causing pain or discomfort, then *rāga* has manifested in us. This suffering (*duḥkha*) is happening because we are attached to a previously experienced pleasure. If we can let go of this attachment, then we can avoid the associated suffering.

Rāga is one of the most powerful causes of suffering and, therefore, one of the most difficult causes to weaken and overcome. It contains within it the fear of not experiencing something again. The word *rāga* can mean "coloring," and an experience can color or leave a stain in our psyche. *Rāga* can arise due to any sensory or emotional attachment. Just as certain colors attract our eyes again and again, sensory pleasures can attract our attention repeatedly until we form an attachment to them. A *rāga* is also like a musical mode that steers our mood, seducing our consciousness into its emotional zone.

When we experience a pleasurable event, a memory is created—one that colors our heart-mind by making us desire that experience again. Each time we repeat the event, the memory is strengthened. The more intense the pleasure, the stronger the memory. This memory can create a habit or addiction, a "pleasure stain" that remains and influences future action.

Our habits or attachments may be stronger than we realize, and they can involve our senses and emotions. For example, a sweet tooth seems mild, yet an attachment to eating sweets can be a very tough attachment to overcome. It can prevent a well-intended weight loss by causing us to eat high-calorie sweets that negate the effects of other dietary improvements. The scent of a cologne, perfume, or essential oil can create attraction, as can simply seeing a beautiful person. Hearing a harmonious melody or angelic voice makes us want to hear more of it. Receiving an extraordinary massage or being touched in a powerful way forms a visceral memory that fuels our desire to feel that touch again.

Strong habits and addictions are even harder to break. An addiction to narcotics or alcohol can cause all kinds of pain and suffering for us and those around us. Behavioral patterns, such as attracting the same kind of personality for a relationship, even though we know that this type of personality is not healthy for us to be around, can also be addictive. Habitual patterns of behavior (*saṁskāra-s*) are formed by *rāga* more than any other *kleśa.*

Rāga is the third *kleśa* and is somewhat parallel to *dveṣa,* the fourth *kleśa.* Both are emotional triggers based on clinging to a past experience. Reducing our involvement with external things (*vairāgya*) counteracts both *rāga* and *dveṣa.* Practicing the tools of *kriyā-yoga* weakens *rāga* and the other psycho-emotional afflictions (*kleśa-s*).

For example, you just ended a passionate but unfulfilling and unhealthy relationship in which you experienced both intense pleasure and pain. It is hard to let go of those experiences and move on with your life. Because the relationship lasted so long, the impressions had time to develop deep patterns in your consciousness (*saṁskāra-s*), which can pull you back into the relationship, despite your mind telling you that going back is not a good idea. It is much more difficult to resist *rāga* and stay away from the person than it is to submit to *rāga* and return to the intense pleasure.

We can apply *kriyā-yoga* in this situation to weaken *rāga*. When we muster the strength to break away from the easy road of following our longstanding tendencies, and we instead listen to our inner voice telling us not to return to the past and to move ahead with our life, then *tapas* is happening. Resisting a powerful habit can be difficult and uncomfortable. *Svādhyāya*, or self-observation, allows us to observe our emotions from a distance and listen to the advice of friends and family. *Īśvara-praṇidhāna* is the letting go of this unhealthy relationship and having faith that life will be OK without it.

Desire is fine as long as we are not attached to its fulfillment. If not being able to reenact a pleasurable experience upsets us, then *rāga* has been activated. Desire is like a fire—it is always burning—and the satisfaction of desires, like the result of any action, must be let go. Our outer wants and ambitions change over time, part of the continuous flux of the universe. Turning our attention inward and experiencing our inner light of awareness naturally diminishes outer desires and cultivates *vairāgya*. Wishing to become better people and improve our lives is healthy and necessary for moving forward on our journey.

THOUGHTS

The need to reexperience an enjoyable
event is a source of suffering.

Past experiences can color present and
future thoughts, words, and deeds.

If I cannot have what I want, I will let go of it and move on.

EXERCISES

To feel how difficult letting go of a seemingly
mild attachment can be, try and abstain from
one of your favorite foods for a while.

Think of a romantic relationship that you wanted to end, but that kept drawing you back in. What made you return? How can you prevent it from pulling you back again in the future?

Have a piece of chocolate. See if you can stop
there and not enjoy another piece.

25

DVEṢA

Clinging to Past Suffering

द्वेष

Clinging to a past that doesn't let me choose.
SARAH MCLACHLAN, from I WILL REMEMBER YOU

LIKE *RĀGA, DVEṢA* IS AN emotional trigger based on clinging to a past experience. When we experience pain or discomfort, it is natural to want to avoid that experience again. *Dveṣa* contains in it the fear of experiencing something again. If an aversion changes our behavior in a way that is not helpful to us, then *dveṣa* is present. Being deliberately cautious because of a prior hurtful event can serve to protect us and, thus, be helpful. When we suffer from resistance, resentment, vengefulness, or anger because of a painful event, then our own consciousness becomes affected in a negative way. Avoiding and hiding the pain of a bad experience represses the emotions, burying them deeper in our consciousness and bodily tissues.

Resistance binds and contracts our energy, stifling openness and change. If we resent another person for saying unkind or untruthful statements about us, *dveṣa* has reared its ugly head. For example, if you heard that a coworker was badmouthing you, instead of resenting him, approach him and kindly ask why he said what he did. Always be aware that miscommunication can create misunderstanding and hurtful thoughts. Allowing any relationship to deteriorate because of festering animosity only brings you down to the level you believe your coworker has stooped to.

The desire to get back at someone is another way *dveṣa* can linger. "An eye for an eye" only hurts, while "Turn the other cheek" promotes compassion and empathy. For example, a long time ago in high school, your girlfriend stole your boyfriend, creating within you a strong sense of distrust, betrayal, and vengefulness. Over the years, you have always wanted to do the same to her. If you succeed, the result will be only more hurtfulness. If you try but do not succeed, the negative energy of revenge will still affect your state of mind. Either way, *dveṣa* is present.

Anger toward someone because of something they did or said affects us more than them. For example, expecting a longtime pessimist to become optimistic, like we are, is unreasonable and bound to result in disappointment. Allowing people to be who they are and where they are is true tolerance. If it is obvious that being around a person is detrimental to our personal growth, then we can minimize our exposure to them until we are strong enough to influence them in a positive way without sacrificing our progress.

A painful trauma often strengthens *dveṣa.* The traumatic experience creates a deep imprint in memory and an automatic aversion to some or all aspects of the event. This imprint (*saṁskāra*) will likely affect how you act in the future, especially when a new situation arises that contains an aspect of the previous trauma. Our heart-mind has been programmed to avoid at all costs anything that might recreate the suffering you went through during the trauma. For example, as a young child, you ran off from your parents' view and were soon surrounded by four barking dogs. Your life seemed threatened, and a deep fear of dogs was instilled in you. Since then, even very friendly dogs scare you. Over time, you can move from extreme caution around dogs to an awareness of when it is OK or not OK to pet a dog. Allowing the trauma to inform better, safer habits and then fade as the new habits strengthen will permit the past event to take its proper place in the present.

Yoga provides techniques to reprogram the heart-mind and root out emotional afflictions such as *dveṣa*. The three practices of *kriyā-yoga* are the most effective way to weaken and eventually eliminate all *kleśa-s*. We can weaken *dveṣa* by first becoming fully aware (*svādhyāya*) of which events trigger our aversion. This self-inquiry can include tracing the negative reaction back (*pratiprasava*) to the event(s) that began this aversion. Talking with long-time friends or with a therapist can assist this process. Then think of a different, positive, and constructive action to replace the unconscious and detrimental reaction whenever the situation arises again.

Implementing this plan (*tapas*) to weaken *dveṣa* is the most difficult part. The next time your aversion begins to arise, step back and do your best to consciously act according to your plan, with faith in its eventual success (*īśvara-praṇidhāna*). It may take several experiences over time to gradually convert the reactive behavior into a helpful and positive pattern.

Sometimes our aversion takes the form of discomfort around certain people, such as immediate family members. Since we are culturally obligated to see family members every so often, we have ample opportunities to work through this particular kind of *dveṣa*.

Every time an aversion erupts is an opportunity to reduce its control of your actions. Future suffering can be avoided if we make a sincere and persistent effort to gain insight into who we really are and how we can consciously act from our divine inner nature, instead of unconsciously reacting based on old, harmful patterns of behavior.

THOUGHTS

A painful experience or trauma is recorded
deep in the subconscious memory.

If I notice when I feel unfriendly or antagonistic,
I can act consciously with kindness instead
of reacting unconsciously with spite.

I will carefully reflect on why I hold an
aversion toward someone or something.

EXERCISES

Are there any foods you disliked as a child and
now avoid? Can you think of a way to prepare
these foods to be appealing to your palate?

Choose a sense (sight, sound, taste, smell, or touch) and
think of an aversion you have related to that sense. Reflect
on how this aversion came to be. Is it good for you or
not? If not, what can you do to weaken or eliminate it?

Think of family members who you dislike, yet have to see once in a while. Make a plan to act toward them in such a way as to reduce their negative effect on you. Instead of avoiding them, seek them out and try out your plan, then experience how your interaction feels compared to previous ones. Keep tweaking your plan until it begins to work.

26

ABHINIVEŚA

Fear of Death

अभिनिवेश

Live your life that the fear of death can never enter your heart.
CHIEF TECUMSEH (CROUCHING TIGER), Shawnee Nation

THE FEAR OF DEATH OR pain exists deep in our subconscious. When we sense that our life is in danger, we fight, flee, or freeze. According to the *sūtra-s*, this primal instinct is embedded "even in the wise," implying it is very, very difficult to overcome. Every species is hard-wired to survive and avoid extinction. It is natural to want to stay alive, yet wanting to stay alive also indicates an attachment to the body.

What is wrong with death? It is a fact of life. Our ego is afraid to let go of our body, mind, habits, possessions, reputation, friends, family, and other fetters of our physical existence, yet once we stop clinging to these things, we become liberated while alive, and death becomes merely a transition from one life to the next. The soul inside, our true essence, never dies.

Abhiniveśa is a deep-seated involvement in the process of dualities, such as pleasure and pain, and an addiction to the game of the *kleśa-s*. Fear is based on attachments such as *rāga* and *dveṣa.* Being caught in the wheel of dualities, we identify with them and see ourselves as a conglomeration of such things as our thoughts, possessions, preferences, and family. Egotism (*asmitā*) keeps us bound to who it thinks we are.

Our state of mind at the time of death contributes to our state of mind in the next life. If the heart-mind imbibes virtue, goodness, and purity at the time of death, then these qualities will carry over into the next life. It is one thing to cultivate an attitude of healing and perseverance in order to survive a life-threatening condition. It is another thing to cling to life, or another's life, when it is not a real life anymore. Accepting death when it is imminent conquers *abhiniveśa* and allows us to move on. The Hindu god of death is named Yama, the same word as the first limb of yoga (which means "regulations, restraints"), because he restrains life itself.

For example, you are traveling on an airplane when all of a sudden the ride becomes rough. You can feel the plane dipping and rising abruptly. How do you feel? What can you do? At that point, you have no control of your fate. The fear of death can only make you worrisome and unhappy. Stepping back and realizing that you have no control (*svādhyāya*) and then surrendering to whatever is going to happen (*īśvara-praṇidhāna*) brings your consciousness back to its center. Mental and emotional calmness ensue in the midst of your chaotic situation. Thus, *abhiniveśa*, our fear of death, is weakened.

Death, like time, exists only in the ever-changing manifest world. That pure light of awareness resting within each of us was never born and will never die; it is perpetual and eternal. As we spend more time experiencing this divine presence and regarding our body as a temporary house for it, our fear of dying lessens. Death becomes simply another change.

Thoughts

Death is not bad. Like life, it is part of
the natural cycle of existence.

When I am in the presence of death, I understand it
to be a positive and necessary transformation.

I will make the most of this life by purifying my
heart-mind and letting go of attachments.

Exercises

Sit in meditation until you are completely disconnected
from the outside world. Who are you now?

Think of a time when you were in a potentially
life-threatening situation. Were you afraid? Why?
What did you learn from that situation?

Pretend you have only one month to
live. What might you do differently?

PART 3

OUTER BEHAVIOR

27

AṢṬĀṄGA

The Eight Limbs of Yoga

अष्टाङ्ग

Practicing the limbs of yoga eliminates impurities
and reveals the light of knowledge, leading to a continuous
and keen sense of discernment.

YOGA SŪTRA 2.28

THE EIGHT LIMBS OF YOGA are a set of practices that develop our civility in society and prepare us for our journey inward to discover our true nature. The deliberate order from outer to inner is consistent with the common textual theme of moving our consciousness from a gross state to a more subtle and refined state. The practice of each limb can occur simultaneously, just as all the limbs of a baby grow at the same time. Implementing all eight limbs into our life virtually guarantees that we will develop into a well-rounded human being. Our inner mind understands who we are and our outer mind acts harmoniously with others.

The eight limbs are the easiest place to begin our journey into yoga. Of all the avenues provided in the *sūtra-s*, they are the simplest to understand and pursue. Each limb is introduced in this chapter, then explored in-depth in the following chapters. The first five limbs are treated as individual "outer" limbs, while the final three "inner" limbs are grouped together in a trio called *saṁyama*, meaning "complete composure." The fifth limb (*pratyāhāra*) occurs naturally as a result of its surrounding limbs and serves as a threshold between outer and inner.

Practicing the eight limbs purifies the body and heart-mind and leads to discriminating perception (*viveka*). Each part of yoga stabilizes and refines a different aspect of our being.

The first limb (*yama-s*) provides guidelines for establishing a strong ethical backbone and, thus, supports the remaining seven limbs.

The second limb (*niyama-s*) consists of personal practices for taking care of ourselves. It includes the components of *kriyā-yoga*, the objective of which is to weaken any negative mental-emotional afflictions (*kleṣa-s*).

The third limb, which is the most well-known and commonly practiced, is *āsana*, which serves to prepare the physical body for seated meditation.

Breath regulation (*prāṇāyāma*) is the fourth limb, serving to remove any obstructions in the flow of our life force.

The fifth limb, tuning out sensory distractions (*pratyāhāra*), naturally occurs as a side effect of breath regulation and the final three limbs—the inner limbs.

The final three limbs are stages of the process of turning inward (*saṁyama*): *dhāraṇā* is choosing and focusing on an object, *dhyāna* is extending the duration of focus, and finally, in *samādhi*, the object receives our complete attention.

The eight limbs of yoga provide a solid framework for living a moral, healthy, and peaceful life. Naturally, our outer thoughts, words, and actions directly affect our inner state and vice versa. Cleaning our sacred body, breath, and heart-mind from the inside out and the outside in, purifies, refines, and prepares us for the ecstatic connection with our divine inner light of awareness, which is our true nature.

THOUGHTS

The eight parts of yoga develop and refine my body, mind, and spirit from the outside in and from the inside out.

I can honor and practice all the limbs of yoga, knowing they will improve the quality of my life.

When I follow the guidelines of yoga, I will become a kind, balanced, and happy person.

EXERCISES

Go through each limb of yoga and write down which of them you practice more often and which you practice less often. Rank the importance of each limb to you.

Think of the limbs you do not practice much. Dedicate some time to them, and think of how you could incorporate them into your life.

If you feel any resistance to the limbs you do not practice, take a moment to examine why.

28

YAMA-S

Ethical Practices

यम

The most important human endeavor is the striving
for morality in our actions. Our inner balance and even
our very existence depend on it. Only morality in our actions
can give beauty and dignity to life.
ALBERT EINSTEIN

OUR WORLD, ESPECIALLY THE MELTING pot of America, is filled with people whose belief systems span the gamut. A civil society functions when all agree on certain basic ethics, called *yama-s* in yoga. The ability to cooperate with others is arguably the most important of the eight limbs of yoga; its importance is emphasized by its placement at the very beginning of the limbs. Social ethics can be practiced more often than the other limbs—in fact, anytime one person interacts with another living being. All other limbs look to the *yama-s* as their foundation.

Social interaction is the best environment in which to ascertain how effective the foundational principles of yoga are. The way we treat other living creatures is a testament to our inner state. Clarity in our heart-mind manifests as qualities such as kindness, compassion, selflessness, and keen judgment. On the other hand, cloudiness reveals itself as malice, selfishness, and poor judgment.

Yama means regulation, control, or restraint. Each *yama* is a guideline for behaving in a benevolent manner toward others so as to support the process of quietly turning inward and discovering our true nature. They are listed below and will be explored in individual chapters:

Yama 1: *Ahiṁsā* (nonviolence)
Yama 2: *Satya* (truthfulness)
Yama 3: *Asteya* (not taking from others)
Yama 4: *Brahmacarya* (conservation of vital energy)
Yama 5: *Aparigraha* (nonhoarding, nonpossessiveness)

The first and foremost *yama* is nonviolence toward other creatures. Truthfulness, when practiced alongside nonviolence, creates a powerful force for goodness in the world. Not taking from others relates to truthfulness in terms of honesty. Conservation of vital energy means practicing moderation by being responsible with our sexual behavior. Finally, reining in the desire to accumulate too many possessions not only helps our environment, but also allows us more time to devote to contemplation and practice.

Each *yama* is considered a great vow, a universal ethic not limited by social class, place, time, or circumstance. Practicing the *yama-s* strictly all the time is possible, but may be too extreme on a practical level. It is up to us to use our discrimination (*viveka*) to determine whether or not observing a *yama* is appropriate.

Practicing all five *yama-s* cultivates a strong moral backbone that will benefit us and others throughout our lifetime. Difficult situations can test our ethical fortitude. The *yama-s* are to be taken seriously and practiced moment to moment. When we maintain our dignity and act truthfully in the face of an ethical challenge, others will follow our brave lead and also behave with a clean conscience.

THOUGHTS

All sentient beings share the same divine inner light.

I can treat others as I would like them to treat me.

I will be kind, honest, not take from others,
be responsible sexually, and not possessive.

EXERCISES

Write down which *yama-s* you feel you could
improve on or practice more in your own life.

Why is *vairāgya*, nonattachment to sensory
objects, important to practicing the *yama-s?*

Think of instances when each *yama* is not appropriate
or when going against one has a benign result.

29

AHIṀSĀ

Nonviolence and Compassion

अहिंसा

It is quite proper to resist and attack a SYSTEM, but to resist and attack its author is tantamount to resisting and attacking oneself. To slight a single human being is to slight the divine powers within us, and thus harm not only that being but with him the whole world.

MOHANDAS K. GANDHI

WHEN WE HARM OTHERS, we harm ourselves, and vice versa. *Ahiṁsā*, which is the first of the five *yama-s*, is the ethical practice of nonhurtfulness toward others and ourselves. It involves abstaining from intentionally inflicting pain on or killing other creatures in thought, word, or deed. A nonjudgmental and forgiving attitude is essential to practicing *ahiṁsā*, the first and most important social observance. *Ahiṁsā* also implies an attitude that strives to reduce harm. All other ethical observances are meant to be practiced alongside *ahiṁsā*. The second one, truthfulness (*satya*), is particularly powerful when observed with nonviolence, since clear and honest communication can prevent misunderstandings that may lead to anger or violence.

Acting against one of the five ethical practices, like resorting to violence, results in endless suffering and ignorance, whether the person performed the action, caused it to happen, or consented to it. If we had our hand in any part of a violent event, then by the law of action-reaction, that energy will come back to us in some fashion. By the law of cause and effect, every action has a consequence.

Greed, anger, and delusion cause us to act unethically. Many innocent people are harmed by someone who will do anything to acquire or maintain power. Sometimes the more money someone makes, the more money he desires, which leads to greediness and a false sense of importance. Then any threat to that person's fortune may cause him to fire someone who works for him or covertly secure the other's exit. Anger contributes directly to violence, such as when a person becomes angry after losing a tennis match and slams her racquet on the court. Delusion can lead to violence as well. For example, when someone laughs while looking at you, you may think she is threatening or mocking you, and you may feel anger and violent thoughts in your heart-mind as a result.

Harming others can occur through thoughts, words, or deeds, each of which we are responsible for. Our state of mind can affect others nearby, and vice versa. A quiet heart-mind calms, whereas an agitated one disrupts. Whenever we direct thoughts toward other people, they receive the energy of those thoughts. For example, looking at someone and thinking to ourselves, "He is ugly," is like saying that thought out loud on a subtle level. Some men will look at a woman with lust in their eyes and minds, and in doing so, make her uncomfortable. On the other hand, thoughts of unconditional love and support will uplift another person. Being considerate by performing acts of kindness stimulates friendship and goodwill among people.

Each person has the potential to be kind or be mean. Practicing the eight limbs of yoga, especially the first limb of ethical behavior, can strengthen our kindness and weaken our meanness. If our kindness is strong enough, we can reduce any meanness we encounter simply by being kind toward it. If, on the other hand, our kindness is weaker than another's meanness, then we may become less kind because of the interaction. In that case, it is better to avoid meanness and be around more kindness in order to strengthen our own kindness. Otherwise, eventually, the meanness will overpower us, and we will become meaner over time. Policemen are especially vulnerable to becoming mean since they interact with violent people on a regular basis.

All sensory information, especially sights and sounds, will influence our heart-mind and create impressions in it. Every time we have an experience, we are colored by it. Therefore, if we want to cultivate nonviolence, we can consciously choose to reduce experiences that expose us to violence, including violent media images, songs, and events, and replace them with positive input that has the character of kindness and compassion.

What do we do if someone is calling us insulting names? Hurtful words have a way of inciting violence. We can let the words pass through us, understanding that the person saying them is unhappy and is directing her frustration toward us. Letting the insults pass may be difficult because the ego may try to identify with and hold on to its interpretation of the words, throwing us into a cyclical whirlpool of negativity. Whatever we convey will eventually return to us. Reacting to negativity by returning the same will only add more harmful energy to the world.

Who suffers when an act of violence takes place? Who benefits from an act of nonviolence? Both parties in both cases. For example, when a bully hits an innocent student, it might feel good to the bully on the outside and make him feel dominant and in control, but inside, he may feel guilty for accosting someone who did nothing to deserve his wrath. Yet that same bully, encountering a person just injured from a car accident, might do what he can to save that person's life, and thus receive a large dose of inner joy in the process.

One antidote to violence, according to Patañjali, is to understand the other side of the story (*pratipakṣa-bhāvana*) and consciously respond in a nonviolent way. If violence is directed toward us, we can use discrimination to determine our response. If we see a violent image or hear angry, hateful words, we can try to remember the opposite, loving-kindness, in order to mitigate the effects of the negative experience.

Ahiṁsā can be applied toward ourselves as well. For example, if you do something wrong, do not beat yourself up about it or regret it for a long time. Be compassionate and kind to yourself, and learn from the experience. Remember, how we treat ourselves will influence our treatment of others.

The practice of nonviolence helps one to rise above the petty game of name-calling, and it can be cultivated in a more skillful way when the ego is under the control of the inner mind, influenced by our pure inner light of awareness. Every time we think, say, or do something harmful to another sentient being, we feel the harm and intuitively know it is wrong. When we notice this behavior, we can apologize or take steps to reverse the negative consequences of this *karma*. *Ahiṁsā* is the key to inner and outer happiness and harmony.

Thoughts

It requires more courage to be nonviolent than
to condone or participate in violence.

I alone am responsible for my thoughts, words, and actions.

I will practice loving-kindness and refrain from harming others.

Exercises

Think of a person whom you often feel negative toward. Send him positive, uplifting thoughts. See if that changes the way you feel around that person.

Have another person say something that normally causes you to react in a negative manner. Try and take a deep breath, then respond in a positive, constructive way.

Think of ways you might be supporting or enabling violence, whether those ways involve interacting with certain people, making particular purchases, or choosing violent types of entertainment. What can you do differently to support nonviolent activities instead?

30

SATYA

Truthfulness and Sincerity

सत्य

The least initial deviation from the truth
is multiplied later a thousandfold.
ARISTOTLE

SATYA, "TRUTHFULNESS," IS THE SECOND of the five *yama-s*. It means communicating what we understand to be true. *Satya* is the *yama* (ethical practice) occurring when our thoughts, words, and actions are consistent with one another. Just as three beams of light shining in the same direction illuminate much better than if they were scattered, so does the combined energy of mind, speech, and action virtually guarantee that the results we expect will happen. Whatever actually exists may differ from what we think exists, which, in turn, may differ from what we communicate as the truth. When our hearts and minds are clean and unbiased, we perceive accurately and communicate clearly.

As a *yama, satya* is second only to *ahiṁsā* (nonviolence). When *satya* is practiced with nonviolence, the remaining *yama-s* and *niyama-s* become much easier. If our thoughts, words, and deeds are harmful, we are not engaging in yoga even though we are practicing *satya.* This is why nonviolence is first among the *yama-s.* Mahatma Gandhi called his nonviolent movement *satya-graha*, meaning "holding to truthfulness." *Satya* and *ahiṁsā* are meant to go hand in hand.

Satya with *ahiṁsā* means clear, honest, appropriate, and helpful communication that considers the short- and long-term consequences. Sensitivity toward others and an unselfish intention for the greater good will likely produce the most positive results. For example, you ask a friend to pick up some bread at the store. If you say, "Pick up some bread," then he will have to guess what kind you want. If you are very specific and say, "I want seven-grain bread made by Sage Bakery," then your communication is clear enough to produce the desired result: the loaf of bread he buys will be what you expect.

Satya also involves a high degree of responsibility and follow-through. If we give our word that we will do something, then it becomes our responsibility to do it. When we follow through on commitments, both we and others grow more and more confident that we will do what we say. On the other hand, if we think one thing and say another, or say one thing and do another, people will question our reliability and trustworthiness.

When thought, word, and deed are the same, they are focused like a laser beam, and our intention is much more likely to come true. Otherwise, if thought, word, and deed are not in alignment, their energies point in different directions and carry much less power, and our expectations are much less likely to come true. For example, you think, "I need to lose weight," and say to yourself and others, "I will lose weight by changing my diet and exercising more." If you follow through with your intention, then you are practicing *satya*, and the results are likely to be what you expect—you will lose weight. On the other hand, if you do not significantly change your diet or lifestyle, your actions are not consistent with your thoughts and words, and the desired result of weight loss will probably not happen.

The media is filled with statements, some true and some untrue. It is our responsibility to separate what is actually true from the falsehoods and deceptions couched as truth. Closer to home, it is just as crucial to evaluate the opinions of family members, friends, and coworkers with whom we interact every day. Be wary of gossip and criticism, and seek out the other side of the story (*pratipakṣa-bhāvana*) before jumping to any conclusions and reacting impulsively. Correct evaluation (*pramāṇa*) is crucial to cultivating truth, and misperception (*viparyaya*) is to be noticed and learned from.

As our field of consciousness clears away the debris of preconceived notions, rigid opinions, and strong patterns of detrimental behavior, we can perceive the outside world as it is and remember events and experiences correctly. Eventually, when what we think matches what is factual, and we communicate the factual thoughts accurately, then *satya* is complete. Speech and mind agree and conform to reality. When our truth aligns with actual facts, then whatever we communicate will be reliable.

THOUGHTS

A clear and compassionate heart-mind
perceives reality as it actually is.

In my search for truth, I can change my mind when
new and sensible information presents itself.

My thoughts, words, and actions will be
consistent, honest, and nonviolent.

Exercises

When do you tend to be inconsistent with your
thoughts/feelings, words, and actions?

Give examples of when:
you thought one thing but said something else,
you said one thing but did something else,
you did something while thinking, "I should not be doing this,"
you did something, then said you did something else (lied),
your memory of what happened or what was
said is different than someone else's.

How do you feel after you have:
lied?
told the truth, even when it was difficult?
pretended you knew something when you did not?
admitted you were wrong?

31

ASTEYA

Not Taking from Others

अस्तेय

The value of a man resides in what he gives
and not in what he is capable of receiving.
ALBERT EINSTEIN

ASTEYA, THE THIRD OF THE five *yama-s* (ethical practices), is not taking from others and accepting only what is earned or freely given. There are many aspects to this ethic, including honesty, trust, generosity, and receptivity.

Asteya shares the principle of honesty with *satya*, the previous *yama*. When our actions show that we are honest, others will trust us. If we know that someone believes in us or is relying on us, we become empowered inside and act to uphold this trust. Being honest and trustworthy contributes to a strong moral backbone as long as our actions remain nonhurtful. All social ethics (*yama-s*) are to be practiced with nonviolence (*ahiṁsā*).

According to the *sūtra-s*, if we do not covet another's property, then more prosperity will come to us. For example, you become a housesitter for a few months. Inside the house are many valuable works of art, pieces of electronic equipment, and so on. If you steal some of these things out of greed or envy, it will ultimately result in future suffering. If you refrain and take care of the house as expected, the owners will trust you and probably have you housesit in the future, allowing you to save money in order to eventually afford your own place.

The opposite of not taking is taking or stealing, which can have many forms. If we interrupt someone during a conversation, we steal their right to be heard. Plagiarizing or taking undue credit for someone else's ideas are also forms of stealing. And, most obviously, stealing something from someone. For example, your server at a restaurant forgot to charge you for something you ordered. If you can muster up the scruples to let the server know, you will see how happy she becomes. On the other hand, if you ignore the mistake and pay less for your meal, you might feel a bit guilty. The choice is obvious if you are keen to develop inner and outer happiness.

A gift is different than an exchange. Offering a true gift means there is no expectation of receiving anything in return. The act of giving alone contains within it the priceless gift of making another feel loved. The holiday of Christmas is supposed to be filled with the joy of giving and be a chance to share with others unconditionally. Often we expect to receive something of equal or greater value than what we give. Giving this way is more of an exchange and can sour a normally joyous holiday with disappointment. The value of a gift lies in the act of giving itself.

Giving without expectation does not always apply in business, where is it commonly understood that the purpose of giving things away is to attain some future benefit. Business is all about trade and exchange, as opposed to true giving. Yet businesses can, for instance, be generous with employee benefits or can give by listening to and addressing staff complaints.

Giving too much can deplete us if we are not receiving at all. For example, social workers give all day, every working day, and need to replenish themselves in order to continue to give. In a personal relationship, it is very important that giving and receiving are in energetic balance. In a traditional role-based marriage, the man provides the material necessities of protection, food, and shelter, while the woman takes care of the house and children. In our modern society, these roles are not as defined. For example, an overly generous supermom or superdad is the primary breadwinner and also takes care of the house and children. Their partner gives little and receives a lot. This gross imbalance fosters resentment and often leads to divorce.

Receiving is giving as well. In many cultures, when food or a gift is offered, acceptance of it is expected and appropriate. This may seem awkward if the giver is living in poverty and the receiver is wealthy, yet by receiving the offering we are honoring the giver's wish. We can use keen discernment (*viveka*) to determine if the giver might expect something in return, or if the gift is way out of proportion to what is appropriate, and then decide whether or not to receive it. Receiving is not as much about the gift as it is about the act of giving. Often it is best to let go and just receive, thereby participating in the continuous flow of the universe.

What is more important, possessing a physical object or knowing how that object affects the heart and mind? When nurturing our inner Self takes priority over satisfying our outer desires, we realize that by giving, we receive, and vice-versa. Shifting the way we think about giving and receiving can transform our consciousness and enable us to avoid future suffering based on expectation. Being generous with others without expecting anything in return nurtures our heart-mind and promotes loving-kindness. Giving is a sacrifice, an offering to another, and a letting go of something. In giving, we open ourselves up a bit and share our heart with another person. Give, and allow yourself to receive.

THOUGHTS

Not coveting or envying what others have
brings gratitude and prosperity.

I can become trustworthy through honesty,
integrity, and contentment.

I will not take what belongs to others or
steal attention away from them.

EXERCISES

Give examples of when:
you took credit for the ideas of someone else,
you gave someone something with expectations
of receiving something in return.

Contemplate yourself: are you more of a giver or a receiver/taker? If you are a strong giver, it may be difficult to receive. The next time someone offers you something appropriate, receive it. If you are more of a taker, find a way to give with no expectation of receiving anything in return.

Think of someone who gives a lot to you or your community. Offer that person a gift in appreciation of her generosity.

32

BRAHMACARYA

Conservation of Vital Energy

ब्रह्मचर्य

It is only when we understand the pursuit of sensation, which is one of the major activities of the mind, that pleasure, excitement, and violence cease to be a dominant feature in our lives.

JIDDU KRISHNAMURTI

YOGA IS CONCERNED WITH CONTROLLING our sensory organs in order to keep us in balance and harmony. Sensual and sexual impulses are powerful forces that are important for us to moderate. We need our sensory organs to live in this world, but when we are attached to these impulses, they become distracting, hijack our attention and use up our life force (*prāṇa*).

Brahmacarya, the fourth of the five *yama-s* (ethical practices), is conserving vital energy, especially sexual energy, in order to channel it in more productive directions. Moving (*carya*) toward supreme truth (*Brahma*) directs the heart-mind away from sensual indulgence, reduces the libido, and thus conserves the sexual fluids that contribute to overall health and vitality. According to Āyurveda, the ultimate product of digestion is the most refined tissue in the body, the reproductive fluids, which fuel *ojas*, the subtle force behind our immune system.

Sexual desire is a powerful force. Regular exercise can be a healthy outlet for some of this energy. Moderation in sexual activity, combined with responsible and appropriate sexual behavior, is an important part of *brahmacarya*. For example, if you are out on a date and your date says she is not ready to spend the night, you must honor her feelings. If you are too attached to your own sexual desires, they can overpower both you and your date. This principle applies even to partners. Loving someone always involves listening to them and treating them as a reflection of yourself.

The opposite, promiscuity or lack of sense control, takes us away from our inner, higher focus and lowers us into the outer world of temporary pleasures and pains. The direction of yoga is toward moderation and balance—enjoying what life has to offer, yet not being attached or addicted to these sensations.

During puberty, *brahmacarya* can be practiced as maintaining celibacy in order to direct hormonal energy into schoolwork. Our budding sexual desire can be ultradistracting and, if not controlled, can derail our education and future. Once we are married or in a committed relationship, *brahmacarya* can be practiced as fidelity, sexual monogamy. Later in life, when we retire and slow down, *brahmacarya* can mean simply conserving our energy. Throughout life, it involves control, moderation, pacing ourselves, and maintaining our inner orientation.

The path of yoga is about living in the outer world responsibly and with kindness, while cultivating a connection with our divine inner Self. Unhealthy attachments and too many external sensory distractions can derail our attention and curtail our progress. Sexual impulses can be toned down by bringing attention to and developing our body, breath, and inner environment.

Controlling sexual and sensual desires so they do not control us is a major step toward becoming a responsible and balanced person, and contributes to lasting inner contentment.

THOUGHTS

Judicious use of sexual energy provides us with the vitality to maintain a healthy body and heart-mind.

I can conserve my vital energy by practicing moderation.

I will strive to channel my vital energy in responsible and appropriate ways.

EXERCISES

Give examples of when:
your sexual desire overpowered and subsumed your studies, work, or thoughts;
you had unmanageable cravings that led to unhealthy habits or behavior.

What have you done in the past to deal with overpowering sexual desires? What worked and what didn't?

What do the words *fidelity* and *celibacy* mean to you?

33

APARIGRAHA

Nonhoarding

अपरिग्रह

It is preoccupation with possessions, more than anything else, that prevents us from living freely and nobly.

HENRY DAVID THOREAU

OUR EGO FEEDS ON GRASPING. The ego constructs our identity and can hold us hostage to our belongings. The ego thinks that we are our body, our mind, and our thoughts and feelings. When it subjugates our inner intelligence, it literally possesses us. As we accumulate material goods, fame, fortune, and so on, our ego becomes stronger. When we step back and realize how shallow these identifications are, that they are based on outer quantities instead of inner qualities, then it is time to reverse our course and turn inward, away from this superficial existence.

Aparigraha, which is the fifth of the five *yama-s* (ethical practices), is not being possessive and applies to material objects, our bodies, and our thoughts. Rejecting the concept of "mine" will be difficult for the ego, but doing so is necessary to progress in yoga. Once we let go of this concept, the *sūtra-s* state that we will understand how we came to be born into this particular life situation. Our current life is a culmination of many births and deaths, all molded by past actions and their impressions (*saṁskāra-s*).

Nonpossessiveness of the heart-mind means not holding on to rigid opinions and not regarding ideas as our own. Whenever we come up with something that appears to be new and original, it is important to realize that we are just tapping into knowledge that already exists (*īśvara*). Our ego loves to hold on to things and call them its own. Our ego loves to call ideas its own and cling to its ideas and opinions. But everything—including the world and ourselves—is always changing, and instead of a rigid ego, we need a flexible heart-mind to navigate these changes comfortably.

Aparigraha also suggests not controlling other people when there is a power differential, such as a boss might try to control her employees, threatening them if they speak up or rock the boat. Hoarding power is a distortion of the ego and always leads to corruption and unethical behavior. *Aparigraha* implies sharing power by listening to other people and acting in a cooperative rather than dictatorial manner.

Money can be used as leverage to control the actions of others. For example, your parents are wealthy, and you are making your way in the world. They may offer to support you in some way in order to covertly exercise some control over your life. There are some people who accept money from a parent, then "allow" that parent to continue to emotionally abuse them. Is the money really worth it? On the other hand, accepting or giving money appropriately, with no strings attached, nurtures our inner conscience, which is a gift far more valuable than any amount of money itself.

As we accumulate stuff, more of our time is spent maintaining it, leaving less time for our own internal development. The "shop till you drop" attitude feeds our bottomless desire to acquire. We are bombarded with advertisements pushing us to buy stuff that we often do not need. We have the ability to rein in this habit of accumulation by carefully deciding to buy only what we will really use and resisting the temptation to purchase impulsively. Less buying means less needs to be manufactured, which reduces our impact on the earth and our environment.

Applied to a conversation, *aparigraha* means allowing others to speak and share their point of view. Dominating a conversation and barely allowing anyone else to chime in is selfish and egocentric. When an extroverted person is talking with a quieter person, it is common for the extrovert to speak most of the time. Partly because our culture is moving so fast, many people feel uncomfortable in an idle moment of silence during a conversation. For the more introverted and quiet individuals, these moments present opportunities to express their thoughts and opinions, which are often quite valuable and insightful. Listening to others, allowing them time to speak, is a form of giving and helps prevent the ego from dominating a discussion.

We are temporary custodians of our belongings. Do they possess us by demanding our time and energy to take care of them? *Aparigraha* involves letting go of attachment to our possessions and not shopping for its own sake. Many people live with so much less than we do. Releasing unused or extraneous possessions to those who need them is an act of kindness and generosity. Lightening our load also frees up time to spend in other ways, especially developing our yoga practice and cultivating a more inward orientation. And the more we experience our pure light of awareness, the less interest we will have in material possessions.

Thoughts

The more stuff we have on the outside, the
less time we have to go inside.

Whenever I give to others, I receive on a deeper, subtler level.

I will lessen my material footprint by acquiring
only what I need or will use.

Exercises

Give examples of when:
you bought something that you only used
once or twice and didn't really need;
you thought of others who needed something
you had, then gave it to them.

Think of ways you can reduce your consumption,
or reuse or recycle what you have.

The next time a moment of silence arises
during a conversation, if you are an:
extrovert, then allow the quieter individuals to say their piece;
introvert, take the opportunity to express yourself.

34

PRATIPAKṢA-BHĀVANA

Cultivating the Opposite

प्रतिपक्षभावन

I have learned silence from the talkative, tolerance
from the intolerant and kindness from the unkind.
I should not be ungrateful to those teachers.
KAHLIL GIBRAN

ALL PEOPLE WANT TO BE heard, understood, valued, and loved. *Pratipakṣa-bhāvana* is the principle of investigating the other side of a story, witnessing an obvious wrong and doing what we can to rectify it, or listening to another's point of view. This practice is most applicable to the five ethics called *yama-s*. Whenever we experience an unethical act or hurtful interaction, it is important to step back and remind ourselves to take the high road, recognizing the inner light of awareness hidden deep beneath another person's thoughts, emotions, habits, and beliefs.

When a falling out occurs between two people, often we hear only one person's rendition of what happened. As a friend or family member, we listen to that person's account and do what we can to support him. Yet we want to avoid generating any negativity toward the other person. When seeking the truth, it is necessary to hear the second person's story as well. Only once we have a complete picture of the events as they unfolded can we clearly discern what happened. It is kind of like being a mediator and listening to both parties before attempting to resolve a conflict. When we are close to one party, it is easy to take that person's side out of loyalty, even when that person may be the cause of the conflict.

For a similar example, when a relationship involving a friend of yours ends, you probably only hear your friend's side of the story, which may make the other person look like the "bad guy." Only when you hear the other person's version of the break-up can you truly understand it yourself. By listening to both sides of the story in a nonjudgmental way, we can maintain a decent relationship with both parties and not run the risk of spreading false information based on one person's opinion. Drilling down to the truth can be difficult and painful. Yet upholding what is right (*dharma*) is part of living according to yoga.

Another meaning of *pratipakṣa-bhāvana* is deciding what to do when we witness an obvious wrongdoing. Actions opposite the *yama-s* are those that are unethical, hurtful, or disturbing. According to yoga, they can be mild, moderate, or excessive, and they come from greed, anger, and delusion. Furthermore, whether such actions are done, approved of, or consented to, they inevitably result in pain (*duḥkha*) and ignorance (*avidyā*). These actions are to be avoided, and when encountered, they may cause us to stand up for what is right.

There are times when we are reminded of what is ethical while experiencing unethical behavior. When we witness events contrary to the *yama-s,* they very well may disturb us. Automatically, we are reminded of opposite, virtuous qualities, like the *yama-s,* and strive to cultivate those instead. Negative thoughts can be used as opportunities to create positive thoughts. In this way, *pratipakṣa-bhāvana* supports the *yama-s.*

If we witness an event that we know is hurtful or unfair, we may be able to intervene to transform it for the better. For example, you see someone shoplifting and become a little uncomfortable. You know in your heart-mind that stealing is wrong; therefore, nonstealing is right. Whether to act or not, and how to act, is up to you, and you must use your discretion to weigh the pros and cons of each possibility.

Pratipakṣa-bhāvana can also mean putting ourselves in another's shoes. Most people act according to habitual patterns based on their past. When we expect other people to act and react just like we do, we are unconsciously projecting our own belief system onto them. Each person has her own unique set of beliefs and characteristics, and each will act according to them. It is essential to try and understand why someone acts the way they do before prematurely reaching a verdict.

In any interaction, remember that you may be entering the situation influenced by your own assumptions, which are based on past experience. A *kleśa* may arise. Before actually doing anything, immediately distance yourself from the resulting emotion that is about to cause a reaction. Then visualize the other side and ask yourself, "How will the other person be affected?" "How much is my own perception of the situation causing this emotion?" At this point, there is opportunity to see what is going on from a more objective vantage point. By acting consciously and compassionately instead of reacting negatively based on our own issues, we build a new, helpful, positive *saṁskāra.*

Pratipakṣa-bhāvana is being aware that there may be another side to every story, honoring other opinions, imagining what it would be like to be in another's position, or acting ethically in the face of injustice. Always striving for the truth, we have the ability and responsibility to understand a situation as best we can and then act in the best interest of everyone.

THOUGHTS

Firm ethical standards and an attitude of fairness give me the strength to counteract negativity.

I can listen to both sides of a story without judging anyone.

I will try to understand each person's point of view and not jump to conclusions based on assumptions or gossip.

EXERCISES

Think of an example of a time when you acted against one of the *yama-s*. Contemplate how you might act if the same event happened again.

Notice the next time you project your own belief system onto someone else. See if you can understand their point of view, and know that they may be projecting onto you as well.

Think of a time when you witnessed someone doing something obviously unethical, and yet you didn't act. Think of another time when you did act. Reflect on why you chose to act or not.

PART 4

PERSONAL PRACTICES

35

NIYAMA-S

Personal Self-Care

नियम

As human beings, our greatness lies not so much in being able to remake the world as in being able to remake ourselves.

MOHANDAS K. GANDHI

THE SECOND LIMB OF YOGA brings our attention to our body and immediate surroundings. The *niyama-s* are like internal (*ni*) *yama-s*. The first limb was about behaving ethically toward others. Now we treat ourselves with care and improve our quality by observing ourselves and implementing changes in our lives that can transform our personality and contribute to our contentment and happiness.

The most external *niyama* is cleanliness, keeping our body, mind, and surroundings free of clutter and impurities. Next is being content with and grateful for who we are and what we have. The final three *niyama-s* compose *kriyā-yoga*, a powerful trio of practices that can be applied every day and that transform our negative habitual patterns into positive action. Each of the *niyama-s* will be discussed in individual chapters.

Niyama 1: *Śauca* (cleanliness of body, heart-mind, and surroundings)
Niyama 2: *Santoṣa* (contentment)
Niyama 3: *Tapas* (practice causing positive change)
Niyama 4: *Svādhyāya* (study by and of oneself)
Niyama 5: *Īśvara-praṇidhāna* (humility and faith)

If we do not take care of ourselves, how can we take care of others? When we are young, we may feel somewhat invincible, thinking that we can do whatever we want to our body and mind without any consequences. As we grow older, we pay the price. For example, college students who drink like fish may end up as alcoholics, or children who grow up eating fast food all the time may end up with Type 2 diabetes.

To live according to yoga, it is our responsibility as individuals to spend time and effort maintaining our body, breath, heart, and mind. Moderation is crucial. It is easy to have lots of fun without trashing your body or mind. Taking good care of our bodies throughout life enables us to avoid much pain and discomfort. A healthy body, with healthy breath, heart, and mind, is a fit vessel for accessing our divine inner light of awareness.

THOUGHTS

Taking care of myself is part of practicing yoga.

When I practice the five *niyama-s*, I begin to self-reflect and learn who I am inside.

A calm, clutter-free environment helps me feel content
and able to commence the practice of *kriyā-yoga.*

Exercises

What do I do now to practice self-care?

How do I feel about my self-care practices? Do they feel like an obligation, or do they give me pleasure?

What other self-care practices would I like to incorporate into my life? Will these be easy to implement? If not, why?

36

ŚAUCA

Cleanliness

शौच

Cleanliness is indeed next to godliness.
JOHN WESLEY

IN THIS ERA OF INFORMATION overload, just keeping up with everything can seem almost impossible. It is easy to live a life that is so busy there is never a moment to slow down and get a handle on everything. Yet taking some quiet time to take care of our body and straighten up our cluttered surroundings will support our progress toward health and clarity. *Śauca*, which is the first of the five *niyama-s*, is the personal practice of maintaining a clean body and clear heart-mind.

Because the physical body is never completely sanitary and requires regular care to keep functioning, it can never be pure. Our body is inherently impure, especially compared to our pure inner light of awareness (*puruṣa*). Our outer, physical shell is like a temple that temporarily houses this awareness. Keeping our temple clean makes it possible to connect with the divine radiance within. The process of yoga is a gradual purification of all layers of our individual self. The physical body is purified through *tapas* and *āsana*, the breath through *prāṇāyāma*, and the heart-mind from all eight limbs of yoga (*aṣṭāṅga*).

Keeping the body clean can remind us of its impermanence, since it is always changing, which in turn can make us realize what does not change and requires no maintenance (the light within). All the stuff we spend time cleaning can also reveal what we are attached to.

Cleanliness can be taken to an extreme if we become uptight when our surroundings are not spic and span all the time. This may be the ego's way of controlling its environment or making up for a deep sense of insecurity from perceived internal impurity. Sometimes a feeling that we are unclean on the inside, often as the result of a past, painful experience, can manifest as obsessive cleaning on the outside. This would be an instance of *dveṣa-kleśa* affecting our actions.

On the other hand, the process of creativity can be stifled by trying to keep everything neat, especially for people who seem to have a perpetually messy work area. All of the thoughts and emotions racing through their consciousness contribute to their creative endeavors. *Śauca* involves allowing the creative process to happen while occasionally stepping back into a quiet space, regrouping our thoughts, updating our to-do list, and organizing our workspace in order to calm the heart-mind and reduce stress and anxiety.

A vegetarian diet aligns with *śauca* since it supports nonviolence (*ahiṁsā*) and promotes *sattva*, that is, qualities such as virtue, kindness, intelligence, and purity. Āyurveda, the Indian science of longevity and medicine, treats all substances objectively, including meat. The lifestyle and diet of yoga promotes eating as low on the food chain as possible. Humans are considered the highest level of consciousness and are also highest on the food chain. Animals are next, then fish, then plants, which are considered the least conscious beings.

"Coming clean" by admitting something that we have been holding in, in order to avoid potential embarrassment, is another form of *śauca.* Expressing deep emotion in a nonviolent way purges the heart-mind of pent up feelings. Mourning the death or suffering of a loved one cleanses our heart-mind as well. Apologizing is extremely cathartic for the heart-mind, while it also weakens egotism (*asmitā-kleśa*).

Outer and inner cleanliness are important for maintaining our health and sanity. *Śauca* leads to a heart-mind that is *sattvic*, happy, focused, not distracted by sensory perceptions, and ready for experiencing the divine light within.

Thoughts

Constant clutter on the outside can indicate continuous chatter on the inside.

Experiencing the unchanging purity of my inner awareness helps me realize the impermanence of my body.

I will keep my body, heart-mind, and surroundings clean and uncluttered.

Exercises

Give examples of times when poor hygiene or disorganization affected your life in a negative way.

Clean off your desk at the office, putting everything neatly in its proper place. This cleaning may be difficult and uncomfortable for you. When you are finished, notice how this change affects your state of mind. Is it more at ease? Quieter? Are you more relaxed?

Think of one food that you know is bad for your body, but that you keep eating anyway. Then think of a possible substitute that tastes just as good, but contributes to your health. See if you can make this replacement temporarily, and then permanently.

37

SANTOṢA

Contentment and Gratitude

सन्तोष

Contentment makes poor men rich.
Discontentment makes rich men poor.
BENJAMIN FRANKLIN

TRUE INNER HAPPINESS RESTS UPON feeling content with who we are right now. Like the rest of the world, we are changing from moment to moment. Possessions flow in and out of our lives, people around us come and go, our opinions and even what we think is true changes over time. Our outer form is in flux around a deeper and permanent light of awareness (*puruṣa*). Complete satisfaction and contentment can be experienced when our heart-mind field of consciousness (*citta*) rests quietly in this awareness.

Santoṣa, which is the second of the five *niyama-s*, is being grateful for what we have and content with who we are and where we are in life. According to the *sūtra-s*, when *santoṣa* is present, unexcelled happiness pervades our being. This feeling of contentment is not the same as what we feel when we have everything we ever wanted in life in terms of possessions, a partner, and an ideal job. Those things can all change. True *santoṣa* comes from the understanding that who we really are at the core is none other than that light of awareness that all beings share.

What satisfies one person does not necessarily satisfy another. It is not fair to project our own means of enjoyment onto other people. For example, some people love to go out to bars and have fun drinking, talking, and dancing. They might think that everyone likes these activities, especially since so many people do them. Yet there are others who do not like doing these things at all and prefer quieter activities, like attending a lecture or class. *Santoṣa* means being satisfied with whatever you are doing, knowing that it, like everything else, will end, and being aware that the eternal divinity within is always present.

The opposite of *santoṣa* is discontent or dissatisfaction, a form of suffering (*duḥkha*). Noticing this feeling is the first step toward converting it. Instead of focusing on what we do not have or why we are not where we want to be, we apply the opposite attitude (*pratipakṣa-bhāvana*) of being grateful for what we have and where we are. As long as we are *doing* something to move ourselves in a positive direction, time and patience will lead us to the desired result. Contentment is not stagnant, because of the changeable nature of our life and the world around us. *Santoṣa* is being aware that we are moving forward and being satisfied with our progress.

How we look in front of others can be another source of dissatisfaction. For example, if we attend a yoga lecture, we may feel we have to sit on the floor, even though doing so is uncomfortable for us, because others are sitting on the floor. Why not just sit in a chair? Even for meditation, it is better to be relaxed and upright in a chair than tense, in pain, and slouched sitting on the floor. When we conform to what we think others expect of us, in order to save face and be accepted by others, we are not content with ourselves.

So often we judge our progress, whether physical, intellectual, emotional, or spiritual, based on comparison with others. Granted, those who have practiced for many years can show us what we may be capable of, but it usually takes time and effort to reach that level. Our culture is used to immediate gratification. Yet a delicious soup results from a long, slow simmer, not a quick and furious boil. So it is with any endeavor, including yoga: the best, most satisfying results come from sincere effort and gradual progress over time. What is important is that we are moving in a positive direction.

Sometimes our progress performing the physical postures, called *āsana-s,* is falsely judged by our level of flexibility. If people can perform all of the "difficult" postures, are they really good at *āsana?* If so, then a ballet dancer or gymnast could walk into a class and be judged the most advanced student. Obviously, this thinking is misperception (*viparyaya*). In fact, even those who are inflexible can be experts in *āsana* if they are exerting sincere effort and understand their bodies and their limitations.

One aspect of contentment is being unattached to the results of our actions. If the result is less than we expected, we can still accept what happens, learn from it, and move on. If we have unreasonable expectations, we may be setting ourselves up for disappointment. For example, you send out an email blast to hundreds of people advertising your new website. When you expect a heavy response, but only 20 percent of your email recipients visit your website, you might become upset. On the other hand, you can be grateful that you received some response and happy that there are people who value your work. A simple shift in the way you think about something can completely transform your attitude toward it. Either way, you will probably begin thinking of ways to make future advertisements more appealing.

If we cultivate gratitude even when we are content, we strengthen that attitude in our heart-mind, like amending its soil, and make that gratitude easier to access when needed. Gratefulness does for our heart-mind what food does for our bodies—it nourishes our heart-mind and creates a sense of fulfillment. Slowing down, stepping back, and appreciating the little things in life creates inner happiness.

Gratefulness is feeling great and full of joy with who we are and what we have. There will always be people with more or fewer possessions than us. Keeping up with the Joneses is an exercise in discontent. Knowing that everyone shares the same divine inner light of awareness can shift our attention away from external material assets and toward the cultivation of our own inner happiness.

THOUGHTS

Feeling satisfied and fulfilled in life
creates deep, inner happiness.

Whether happy or despondent, I can
feel grateful for what I have.

I will set reasonable expectations and
fully accept whatever happens.

EXERCISES

Give examples of when you tend to be dissatisfied, wanting results to be different than they turn out to be.

The next time you are waiting for something you did not expect to wait for, find a way to enjoy that precious idle time.

Ponder all that you have to be grateful for, such as health, friends, community, and life. Think of the millions of people around the world who have so much less in comparison, yet are happy nevertheless.

38

KRIYĀ-YOGA

Practice in Action

क्रियायोग

A journey of a thousand miles begins with a single step.
CONFUCIUS

REAL INNER TRANSFORMATION CAN OCCUR when we deliberately investigate why we act or react the way we do. Understanding what our longstanding behavioral patterns are and what caused them in the first place provides the opening we need to change the ways we think and act. This practice of self-transformation could be the most difficult part of our journey through yoga. Faith in ourselves and in the universe supporting this endeavor will allow the process to bear fruit.

Kriyā-yoga, defined by Patañjali as the last three personal practices (*niyama-s*), is a set of synergistic tools that bring about inner change. It consists of *tapas, svādhyāya*, and *īśvara-praṇidhāna. Tapas*, practice causing positive change, involves conscious and deliberate action. It is the most outer, external practice and, thus, is first in the list. *Svādhyāya*, observation by and of oneself, allows us to see what aspects within us need improvement. *Īśvara-praṇidhāna* keeps us humble and respectful by honoring knowledge itself, while providing us with the confidence that positive change will happen over time. These last three *niyama-s* will be discussed in individual chapters.

When these three are practiced in collaboration, the triad becomes a powerful mechanism for learning and growth. *Kriyā-yoga* is one of the easiest systems to understand, yet quite difficult to implement since it involves real, on-the-ground change to our personality. It is a simple, straightforward formula to engage in if practiced with great tenacity and purpose. Since each component informs the others, change is more profound and noticeable when they are practiced together.

Kriyā-yoga is the seed for the eight limbs of yoga (*aṣṭāṅga-yoga*). The threefold set of tools is to be integrated into the other practices. Inner growth involves changing the way we look at things, the way we operate, and our attitudes and expectations. Applying *kriyā-yoga* to our life is easiest if we begin with self-observation (*svādhyāya*) and then carry out a plan (*tapas*) with faith and humility (*īśvara-praṇidhāna*).

The purpose of *kriyā-yoga* is twofold: to weaken our mental-emotional afflictions (*kleśa-s*) and cultivate complete attention (*samādhi*). The practices of *kriyā-yoga* cause our reactions to previously uncomfortable or painful events to diminish, eventually transforming them into conscious and positive actions because the events no longer push any of our buttons. This transformation clarifies and purifies our heart-mind field (*citta-prasādana*), allowing us to focus our attention fully and perceive things as they are.

Thoughts

Diminishing inner pain requires proactive change, self-observation, and acceptance of progress.

I want to improve my well-being through deliberate and lasting inner transformation.

When I practice *kriyā-yoga,* I weaken the root causes of suffering and calm my heart-mind.

Exercises

Which of your current practices support positive change in your life?

Choose an area of your life that you'd like to improve, and observe yourself. For instance, if you are impatient, observe yourself waiting in a long line, and notice your reactions. Is there any way you can work on this area of your life to transform it in a positive way?

Think of all the ways that you have acquired knowledge in your life, whether through your parents, your friends, your teachers, or the natural world. Express gratitude to these people and things that have expanded your world.

39

TAPAS

Practice Causing Positive Change

तपस्

Make a change.
Feel the heat of resistance
melt away old habits
and burn through ruinous conditioning.
Offer negative behavior
into the fire of *tapas*
and chart your course toward freedom.
NICOLAI BACHMAN

THE PRACTICE OF YOGA IS part of a long and gradual process of deliberate external and internal transformation. *Tapas*, which is the third of the five *niyama-s* (personal practices), is the practice of actually implementing our plan for self-improvement. The word *tapas* derives from *tap*, meaning "to heat." Real and permanent change in behavior creates heat from the friction of a new, positive pattern rubbing up against an old, negative one. This priceless heat of discomfort is the result of *tapas*. It can arise while we are exercising (such as during yoga *āsana*), breaking an old habit, changing our direction in life, or doing any other activity that causes positive change. The heat generated by practicing *tapas* will incinerate physical, mental, and emotional impurities, and refine the body, sensory organs, and heart-mind.

Tapas, along with self-observation/study (*svādhyāya*) and faith/letting go (*īśvara-praṇidhāna*), makes up the yoga of action (*kriyā-yoga*), a powerful triad of tools for weakening our mental-emotional afflictions (*kleśa-s*) and moving toward complete attention (*samādhi*).

Change is an inevitable quality of nature (*dṛśya*), and stagnation goes against nature's ebb and flow. In our body, muscles tighten up, opinions become rigid, and habits solidify. *Tapas* causes heat and thus change, and therefore can prevent obstructions from forming in our body, breath, and heart-mind. One of the most common forms of *tapas* is doing a sequence of postures (*āsana-s*) with enough effort to release heat by stretching and strengthening the muscles in the body.

Habitual behavior causes stagnation. When we consciously change a habit, discomfort (*duḥkha*) arises and creates heat in the body. This is the priceless heat of real change. If we are aware that the discomfort is good for us, it becomes a desirable effect and may encourage our continued practice. *Tapas* includes consciously challenging long-standing patterns of behavior (*saṁskāra-s*), and gradually burning them up, resulting in spiritual and physiological growth. Opening up to new ideas and behaviors also creates heat as the circuits in our brain are rewired.

For example, think of a strong habit, some action that you have done the same way for many years—let's say the way you brush your teeth. Try and brush them using the opposite hand, or moving the brush through your mouth in a different sequence. This change will feel uncomfortable at first, but with enough repetition a new pattern (*saṁskāra*) will form, and the movement will become easier. Next, try choosing a habit that you know is obstructing some aspect of your life. Set an intention and make a commitment to change the habit. An attitude of *satya* will help you follow through with your plan.

A traditional, orthodox view sees *tapas* as an austere practice of enduring physical pain in order to become detached from the mortal body. One such practice is called *pañcāgni*, meaning "five fires," where a person sits in the hot sun (fire number one) surrounded by four fires and tries to meditate. This kind of ascetic practice may have merit in a different culture, time, or place, but in contemporary Western society, it may not be appropriate. The idea is to become impervious to the pairs of opposites, such as heat and cold, wet and dry, that assail the sensory organs and draw the attention outward toward external objects. Any *tapas* that is harmful to ourselves or others violates the principle of *ahiṁsā* (nonharming).

Tapas requires discipline and effort. In Indian lore, a sage would practice *tapas* and celibacy for thousands of years to accumulate lots of power. When the gods noticed that their power was threatened, they sent down to earth a beautiful nymph who tried to distract the sage from his meditation. If she succeeded in seducing him, he would lose his seed and, thus, his power (see chapter 32, *Brahmacarya*).

In yoga, healthy change is necessary for progress to occur. After setting an intention to commit to positive changes in your life, formulate specific actions to take or ways you wish to respond when certain buttons are pushed. Then, with discipline and effort, implement the plan and burn through the negative, harmful patterns. The inevitable pain or discomfort (*duḥkha*) will produce the sweet nectar of positive, lasting inner transformation.

THOUGHTS

Yoga practice purifies the body, refines sensory awareness, and clarifies the heart-mind.

The discomfort I feel during the process of growth and transformation is necessary and beneficial.

I will practice with a motivation to burn up bodily impurities and welcome positive change.

EXERCISES

Select a mild habit, like eating the same breakfast every day or mowing the lawn in the same pattern every time, and change it for one or two days. Notice how that change feels. Refreshing? Uncomfortable? Difficult?

The next time you exercise, which may be an *āsana* practice, push yourself just a little bit more (without risking injury) and feel your muscles and fascia opening and generating heat. This is the heat of *tapas*.

Think of a person who is difficult, but necessary for you to interact with. Even if you do not like the person, see if you can maintain a positive and kind attitude toward her, especially when the person says words that you would normally react to in a negative way. After the interaction, reflect on how you felt as it was happening. Did you heat up? Did the kindness cool down the dynamic between the two of you?

40

SVĀDHYĀYA

Study by and of Oneself

स्वाध्याय

Sometimes you study the way by casting off the mind.
Sometimes you study the way by taking up the mind. Either way,
study the way with thinking, and study the way not thinking.

EIHEI DOGEN

THE FIRST STEP TOWARD self-improvement and self-refinement is looking at ourselves honestly and objectively. Learning about ourselves and our relationship to the outside world can provide us with a glimpse of who we are. Close friends can act as clear mirrors, revealing shortcomings otherwise invisible to our own perception. Studying sacred books and repeating powerful words or sounds will broaden our understanding of ourselves and others. We may or may not like what we discover.

Svādhyāya, which is the fourth of the five *niyama-s* (personal practices) is learning about and developing the heart-mind (*citta*) by reading and listening to promote self-reflection, by reciting mantras, and by observing ourselves in action. Looking at ourselves insightfully brings us awareness of our strengths and shortcomings. Once we understand where we are, we can set an intention to let go of our negative qualities and reinforce those that have a positive effect. *Svādhyāya* includes understanding our physical, mental, and emotional bodies; our actions and impressions (*karma-s*); and the world around us.

Svādhyāya, along with *tapas* and *īśvara-praṇidhāna*, compose *kriyā-yoga*, a powerful triad of tools for weakening the *kleśa-s* and realizing *samādhi* (complete attention/absorption). *Tapas*, practice causing positive change, naturally leads to *svādhyāya* as we observe the changes happening and adjust our practice or behavior to maintain our desired direction. *Tapas* informs *svādhyāya* and vice versa. Practicing *tapas* often involves resisting the urge to act according to our habitual tendencies. This resistance may heat us up during the course of the interaction. Afterward, we might wait until the heat diminishes, then, in a quieter space, reflect back on that experience of *tapas*.

For example, you notice how frustrated you become when you have to ask your child to brush her teeth many, many times before she does so. This frustration can cause you to become angry toward the child and maybe raise your voice at her, especially if the two of you are under pressure to be somewhere by a certain time. Afterward, you reflect on the interaction and try to think of ways to avoid becoming angry. Eventually, after trying many different techniques, you come upon one that works and is in accordance with the ethical practices (*yama-s*).

During the practice of self-observation, we can ponder what causes us and those around us suffering by asking ourselves: In what situations do I react, and why? How much of my response is automatic, controlled by my past (*rāga* and *dveṣa*)? What are my habitual tendencies (*saṁskāra-s*)? How do my actions or reactions affect the outcomes? How can I convert negative outcomes to positive outcomes?

Traditionally, *svādhyāya* meant learning and repeating a mantra chosen by our teacher for us and studying sacred texts that guide us inward, like the Veda-s, Upaniṣad-s, or Bhagavad-Gītā. The mantra *Om* is the most common mantra, and its repetition connects us with *īśvara*. If we have chosen a deity to relate to, then a mantra to that deity activates the energetic link between us and it. For example, the Hindu god Gaṇeśa represents the energy of abundance and the clearing away of obstacles. Chanting a mantra specifically to Gaṇeśa will connect us to that energy and help bring it into our life.

Studying ancient scriptures is helpful if they are meaningful to us. Since the texts of most religions were written long ago in a language foreign to most of us, we may need to seek out a worthwhile and relevant translation and interpretation of our chosen scripture. We can also study books or listen to audio recordings that cause us to ponder our nature or our surroundings, that lead us to improve ourselves in some way, or that help us to refine our yoga practice. Selecting a valid source of knowledge (*pramāṇa*) requires keen discernment (*viveka*).

Keeping a daily diary of actions that we were not proud of is extremely beneficial since it brings awareness to parts of ourselves that we can improve. Rereading our diary may reveal patterns of behavior, providing a key to unlocking their original causes. Journaling regularly allows our daily thoughts and feelings to be expressed on paper, an exercise that in and of itself teaches us about who we really are.

Through *svādhyāya* it is possible to understand anything about ourselves. Self-observation is the key to understanding who we truly are. When followed through (*tapas*) with faith and humility (*īśvara-praṇidhāna*), self-observation gives us the power to convert old, harmful behavior into new, helpful action. The ultimate goal is complete self-knowledge, with the realization that we are a changing outer shell surrounding a pure, unchanging, inner light of awareness.

THOUGHTS

Recitation of a mantra will connect me with
my chosen form of divine energy.

Sacred and uplifting study contributes to my
personal growth and improvement.

I will take time each day to reflect on my
thoughts, words, and actions.

EXERCISES

Sit quietly and ponder yourself deeply. Write down those areas of your practice or behavior that you feel need improvement or refinement. These can be areas such as eating patterns, discomfort around certain people, or ways you react to certain situations. Think of different courses of action that will promote a positive outcome, making sure they are nonhurtful, truthful, maintain healthy boundaries, and understand the point of view of the other person, if there is one involved.

Begin keeping a daily diary. At the end of each day, recollect the situations in which you behaved positively and those in which your behavior was detrimental.

Find a book or audio recording that helps you discover more about yourself. Make sure its viewpoint is not hurtful or critical toward anyone and includes tolerance for other belief systems.

41

ĪŚVARA-PRAṆIDHĀNA

Humility and Faith

ईश्वरप्रणिधान

Faith is an oasis in the heart which can never be reached
by the caravan of thinking.
KAHLIL GIBRAN

IF OUR QUEST FOR KNOWLEDGE is confined to what our intellect can understand, then we will never experience the deepest and subtlest aspects of ourselves. Logic works well in the outer world of names and forms, but breaks down as our focus turns inward. Faith in something beyond our limited self is essential to circumventing linear, logical thought. Letting go of our past conditioning allows us to perceive the material world without the fetters that bind us to it. The practice of *īśvara-praṇidhāna*, which is the fifth of the five *niyama-s* (personal practices), bypasses these distractions through faith and surrender to something higher than ourselves, thereby eliminating egotism and cultivating humility.

Belief in a power higher and more subtle than ourselves is fundamental to most religions. The worldview of yoga includes belief in a universal source of knowledge (*īśvara*) that is not bound by anything, and an individual inner light of awareness (*puruṣa*) that resides in the body and is exposed to our perceptions, actions, thoughts, and emotions. *Īśvara-praṇidhāna* is the personal practice (*niyama*) of deep respect for, admiration of, and faith in a higher, inner knowledge. A clear and receptive heart-mind promotes insight into this omniscience. *Īśvara-praṇidhāna*, along with *tapas* and *svādhyāya*, compose *kriyā-yoga*, a powerful triad of tools for weakening our negative patterns of behavior and realizing *samādhi*.

Īśvara-praṇidhāna cannot happen if doubt is present. Doubting ourselves is an obstacle (*antarāya*) to yoga and will make faith impossible. Doubt can spoil any chance of success. True faith and surrender bypass the heart-mind and connect us directly with the object of devotion. To be successful, there can be nothing in the way.

Faith in the unknown can neutralize fear of the unknown. As it is said, "Attitude is everything." It is better to project the positive energy of optimism and faith than to expect and fear the worst. Faith is what allows us to release our attachments to the results of our actions, thus freeing us from the potential disappointment—the suffering—that can arise when results don't match our expectations. When we have faith in a higher power, we accept that whatever happens as a result of our action is exactly what is meant to happen, even if it doesn't match what we expect.

We can let go of our attachments and expectations by understanding the transient nature of all things, stilling our heart-mind (*nirodha*), and listening to our inner teacher. Action based on inspiration and not bound by expectation is truly free. Dedicating the fruits of our actions to *īśvara* allows us to let go of them.

According to the *sūtra-s*, the practice of *īśvara-praṇidhāna* leads to the attainment of *samādhi*. A superficial, egoic view of the outside world sees us as separate and distinct from other things. Yoga as *samādhi* is the subtle state of mind in which we experience an external object as no different than ourselves. We seem to join with our object of focus. When the ego relinquishes control, allowing the heart-mind to reflect the object like a mirror, then the subject (the mirrorlike heart-mind) looks exactly like the object. When we can fully surrender to a higher power, the unconditional devotion (*bhakti*) bypasses any other distracting thoughts and emotions (*vṛtti-s*), rendering them quiet (*nirodha*) and leading to the state of *samādhi*.

Cultivating a heart-mind that sees the divine energy inside each person is the practical culmination of this *niyama*. Perceiving no difference between ourselves and others cuts through unawareness (*avidyā*), demotes egotism (*asmitā*), and is a form of *samādhi*. Pure love is independent of the outer, changing world around us. When we understand that each person is a constantly changing outer shell encasing an unchanging, pure inner light of awareness, then we can show love for the divine in all sentient beings.

Praṇidhāna implies a state of humility in the presence of something higher. We all have limitations, yet share the uniquely human ability to self-reflect and the capacity to experience something beyond our conditioned heart-mind. The words *namaḥ te*—which combine to form *namaste*, a common greeting in India—literally mean "salutations to you" and imply "salutations to the divine within you."

Humility means that egotism (*asmitā-kleśa*) is not active and that anything the ego thinks it owns can be passed through us to our teacher or to the universe. For example, if you think that what you teach or purport belongs to you, then *asmitā-kleśa* has reared its possessive head. Any teaching that you think is uniquely your own is the result of an integration and extrapolation of past learning and experience. Let the accolades coming toward you pass right through by honoring, respecting, and giving credit to your past teachers and to teachings that have contributed to your unique way of transmitting useful information.

Serving others is serving *īśvara*. If the results of and credit for all actions are offered to *īśvara*, then our ego cannot hold on to anything, egotism (*asmitā*) weakens, and we receive because of our giving. Having faith in the law of *karma* (what you sow, so you will reap) will encourage thoughtfulness and love toward others. For example, you decide to help feed the homeless one night at a soup kitchen. This act of selflessness nurtures your spirit; you subtly receive on the inside by giving on the outside.

No matter who we are, no matter what our station in life, no matter how much or how little money we have, each of us has the ability to act with humility and trust that whatever happens, happens. *Īśvara*, the source of knowledge, exists for us to learn from, aspire to, and revere. May we dedicate all endeavors to *īśvara*.

THOUGHTS

No one owns knowledge. We all dip into the giant soup of universal intelligence.

Surrendering to the divine allows me to truly understand my relationship with it.

I will give credit for all that I accomplish to my teachers and to the teachings themselves.

Exercises

Get together with a friend and have that friend flatter you. Each time you receive the flattery, notice how you feel and how you respond. Is it inflating your ego too much? Can you feel good about yourself while still letting go of it? Where can you redirect the accolades? How does this redirection change your response?

Think of something that a person close to you says that really bothers you. Have a friend pretend to be that person and say the same thing to you. How does hearing those words make you feel? Why? How can you respond in a kind yet constructive manner, always distinguishing between their inner spirit and their accumulated patterns?

Practice letting go of attachment to an expectation. For example, you bought tickets to a concert that you were really looking forward to. On the way, you get a flat tire. Will you curse till the cows come home, or accept what happened and let go of your attachment to attending the concert? Which action is better for your own peace of mind?

42

ĀSANA

Refinement of the Body

आसन

There is a road in the hearts of all of us,
hidden and seldom traveled, which leads to an unknown,
secret place. To sit or lie upon the ground is to be able to
think more deeply and to feel more keenly.

CHIEF LUTHER STANDING BEAR

YOGA IS MUCH MORE THAN performing physical postures. Yet doing these postures (*āsana-s*) purifies and prepares our body for seated meditation. Our physical health affects our heart-mind and vice versa. As we twist, jump, stretch, and invert all parts of our physique, impurities are churned up and released, allowing our life force (*prāṇa*) to flow more easily and improving our overall well-being.

Āsana is the third of the eight limbs of yoga (*aṣṭāṅga*). The word *āsana* means "sitting" or "seat." *Āsana* precedes breath regulation (*prāṇāyāma*) because *āsana* works on the outer, physical layer of our being, while *prāṇāyāma* works with our breath (*prāṇa*), an inner and more subtle layer of our being. The body needs to be strong and pliable to ground the *prāṇa* flowing through its subtle energy channels. The aim of *āsana* is to reduce any hyperactivity in the nervous system and prepare the body for *prāṇāyāma*. If one cannot sit still comfortably with the spine erect, the *prāṇa* cannot flow unobstructed. On the other hand, it is important to be able to breathe consciously during the practice of *āsana*, so they work hand in hand.

Patañjali does not emphasize *āsana* and devotes only three *sūtra-s* to it, just enough to mention the basic characteristics of its practice. The Yoga Sūtras treats *āsana* as a small but important step along the path of yoga. There are other texts that go into much more detail about *āsana-s*, including what they look like and how to perform them.

When sitting in meditation, we should feel stable and comfortable. Feeling stable means not moving, not teetering, not fidgeting at all. Feeling comfortable implies feeling no pain or anxiety, being relaxed and at ease. These two qualities can be achieved when there is no more exertion and the body is able to sit upright while completely relaxed. Sitting on a chair may be required if the body is not yet flexible enough to sit this way on the floor. Many practitioners feel the need to sit on the floor for meditation, but if discomfort is present, it will defeat the purpose. It is perfectly fine to sit in a chair until our *āsana* practice has prepared us to sit on the floor.

On the other hand, when our attention is focused completely, then we are no longer affected by our surroundings, like heat and cold, pleasure and pain. There are some practices that encourage sitting uncomfortably and in pain, so our heart-mind can work through these distractions, eventually becoming so focused that it is able to ignore them. When we can sit effortlessly still and relaxed regardless of whether or not there are distractions, with our heart-mind focused on the infinite within, then the *prāṇa* is stable and *pratyāhāra* occurs naturally, leaving us undisturbed by sensory stimuli.

Āyurveda is yoga's sister science of health and medicine, and its principles, practices, and goals go hand in hand with those of yoga. If the body is not properly cared for, then the breath and heart-mind will be adversely affected, making it very difficult for us to focus inward and connect with our true nature. Disease is an obstacle to yoga (*antarāya*) and, therefore, is to be prevented whenever possible. *Āsana* is the exercise aspect of Āyurveda. A poor diet or stressful lifestyle will work against our *āsana* progress. It is important that all aspects of our life be in alignment for us to achieve the maximum benefit.

Āsana can be extended to mean our inner posture, our poise, during interactions with others. We want a balance of open-mindedness with groundedness. Being too rigid with our opinion may indicate an attachment to something and is likely connected to egotism (*asmitā*). Closed-mindedness is an aspect of ignorance (*avidyā*). On the other hand, we may have no opinion about anything and go along with whatever anyone says. Our heart-mind may be weak and lack the strength to take a stand. Apathy, an obstacle to yoga (*antarāya*), may also be present; we simply do not care about what is being discussed, even if it is very important. Yoga involves independent thinking—forming our opinions based on as much reliable information (*pramāṇa*) as possible. Following others blindly is another form of ignorance (*avidyā*).

The practice of *āsana* purifies the body and clarifies the heart-mind. Our body is a sacred temple designed to make it possible for us to self-reflect and connect with a higher awareness within. When our limbs are supple, our breath is smooth, and no energy is blocked, we can relax and focus our attention inward, cultivating inner beauty and happiness.

THOUGHTS

A relaxed body and focused heart-mind bring stability and ease.

Yoga postures can transform the state of my body and heart-mind into one that is finer and subtler.

I will balance flexibility with firmness in all aspects of my life.

EXERCISES

If you are not comfortable sitting on the floor for meditation, try sitting in a chair. See if you are able to relax more while still keeping your torso from slouching.

When sitting for meditation on the floor, notice what hurts (like your hips or knees). Find out what specific postures will help you sit without pain. Then give emphasis to those postures in your practice.

The next time you are in a conversation with others, notice which of your opinions may be too rigid or too loose. What can you do to balance those?

43

PRĀṆĀYĀMA

Regulation of Breath

प्राणायाम

A healthy mind has an easy breath.
ANONYMOUS

STABILIZING AND REFINING *PRĀṆA*, our life force, is the centerpiece of yoga practice. As the fourth of the eight limbs, *prāṇāyāma* is where we begin to work with our subtle body via the breath. *Prāṇa*, equivalent to *chi* in Chinese, is responsible for all movement in the body and directly influences our physical, mental, and emotional health. When *prāṇa* flows smoothly, our attention can focus and our heart-mind can calm down.

Life itself is defined by the existence of *prāṇa;* the word *prāṇa* means "life force" or "breath." When a baby is born, everyone waits for its first breath or utterance, an indication that its individual life (apart from the mother) has begun. After a person's last breath, *prāṇa* leaves the body at the time of death. One is not declared dead until the heart stops, the breath stops, and the pupils of the eyes are dilated and unresponsive. These symptoms indicate there is not enough *prāṇa* in the body to sustain life.

Prāṇa is the energetic link that carries sensory information in and action impulses out of the human system. *Prāṇa* moves everything in the body, including blood, lymph, nerve impulses, and ions. It also moves within our subtle energy points (*marma-s*), energy channels (*nāḍī-s*), and energy centers (*cakra-s*).

The mind influences the body, and vice versa, through the *prāṇa* flowing in the nervous system, the breath, and the subtle energy channels. Wherever the mind goes, the *prāṇa* follows. In other words, wherever our attention is directed, our life force is projected. This means that our thoughts can affect our body via the nervous system. Studies have shown that the power of a focused mind, through visualization or a complete shift in attitude, can significantly alter the course of disease. If we can control our life force, we can improve our overall health and well-being.

Prāṇa can even emanate from the body when we concentrate our attention. Thoughts are considered to be waves of *prāṇa* that have an ever so subtle effect on their destination. For example, I have noticed that when my daughter is sleeping and I think about her waking up, she stirs in her sleep. You may have experienced someone turning their head toward you after you have been looking at them from a distance, trying to get their attention.

Breath is a physical manifestation of *prāṇa*, the life force that connects all aspects of perception. When the life force is obstructed, the breath becomes irregular. For example, when we are frightened, our *prāṇa* is shocked, causing us to gasp. If we are stressed, taking a few deep breaths relaxes our body and calms our mind.

Prāṇāyāma calms the nervous system by means of breathing exercises that control and regulate the breath. Irregular breathing patterns and restlessness indicate blockages to the flow of *prāṇa* and result from the nine obstacles to practice (*antarāya-s*). *Prāṇāyāma* balances and slows down the breath, which helps to clarify the heart-mind (*citta-prasādana*) and prepare it for the journey inward (*saṁyama*). *Prāṇāyāma* comprises both the practices involving the breath and the resulting breath regulation and control. Breathing exercises manipulate the *prāṇa* and directly affect the body and the mind through the nervous system, so they have the potential to be very helpful or very harmful. It is safest to learn *prāṇāyāma* from an experienced teacher.

According to the *sūtra-s*, there are three primary *prāṇāyāma* activities: exhalation, inhalation, and retention. Exhalation is relaxing, inhalation is stimulating, and retention is neither. Each activity is done a certain number of times, for a certain duration of time, with our attention directed toward a certain location in the body. The goal of *prāṇāyāma* is to have our breathing become smooth as silk, with no blips.

There is a fourth activity of *prāṇāyāma*, which is really inactivity: stillness of the breath, as if the air in the lungs were passively mixing with the air outside. This state occurs during the practice of *saṁyama*.

Prāṇāyāma, through its effects on the physical body and the mind, helps stabilize and calm them. Practicing this part of yoga helps us bring our attention away from sensory stimuli (*pratyāhāra*) and toward a point of focus. From there, we turn inward, practicing the inner limbs of yoga (*saṁyama*), and gradually experience more and more of a connection with that divine inner light of awareness that rests inside of our core.

THOUGHTS

When *prāṇa* flows quietly, evenly, and unimpeded, we are able to focus, and our inner light is revealed.

I can ascertain the irregularities in my breathing and take steps to even them out.

I will recondition my breathing until it becomes long, smooth, and subtle.

EXERCISES

During your *āsana* sequence, pay attention to your breath within each posture. Notice if there are any irregularities and in what positions they occur.

Sit quietly and follow your breathing pattern. Notice how easy it is to change your breath. See if you can breathe with as little movement as possible.

Seek out an experienced teacher of *prāṇāyāma* and study under their guidance.

PART 5

INNER DEVELOPMENT

44

PRATYĀHĀRA

Tuning Out Sensory Input

प्रत्याहार

The inner gate opens only when the outer gates are closed.

HAZUR

WHEN WE FOCUS OUR ATTENTION on a single thing, all other commotion around us seems to fade. As we go inward toward self-knowledge, we naturally turn away from and let go of outer attachments. During the shift from an outer orientation to an inner one, our senses become sharper and more controllable. As our heart-mind approaches complete attention (*samādhi*), outer and inner distractions cease.

Pratyāhāra is the fifth of the eight limbs of yoga (*aṣṭāṅga*); it is also the last of the "outer limbs" and the pivotal juncture between outer and inner. It is considered an outer, external limb only because it involves the sensory organs. *Prati* means "against," and *āhāra* means "that which is ingested." So the word *pratyāhāra* literally means "opposed to ingestion." *Pratyāhāra* prevents sensory perceptions from entering our field of consciousness.

Pratyāhāra is not a practice per se, but a side effect of breath regulation (*prāṇāyāma*) and turning inward (*saṁyama*).

Prāṇāyāma serves to slow and smooth out the breath, a prerequisite for being able to focus the attention. When our attention is inwardly concentrated (*saṁyama*), we do not register sights, sounds, or other sensory details around us and are no longer distracted by external objects. Therefore, our senses are, essentially, turned off. The sensory organs now follow the heart-mind instead of the heart-mind catering to external sensory distractions. Sensory perceptions, food of the outer mind, are not ingested and, therefore, do not cause any reaction or disturbance in the heart-mind.

There is a metaphor in the Katha Upaniṣad involving a chariot being driven down a road. The road represents sense objects, things we see, hear, touch, smell, or taste. The horses represent our sensory organs, and the reins symbolize our outer mind. The chariot driver symbolizes our inner mind. The driver uses the reins to direct the horses just as the inner mind uses the outer mind to interact with the sensory organs. The chariot master, our inner light of awareness (*puruṣa*), guides the driver. The driver letting the horses out of his control reflects our heart-mind being controlled by our senses and the objects they are attracted to. With no guidance, our senses will carry our attention outward, like horses running wild. Humans are considered to be highly evolved animals who have the ability to act consciously, not just instinctually. When our discerning intellect (the driver) listens to the higher Self (the master), the intellect can guide the outer mind (the reins) in the desired direction, and the sensory organs (the horses) will follow. *Pratyāhāra* results in complete mastery over our sensory organs, a prerequisite for fully connecting with our inner light of awareness.

In the Bhagavad-Gītā, Arjuna (representing a human) has a conversation with Kṛṣṇa (representing his inner, higher Self) and experiences the universal struggle between spiritual development and sensory indulgence. Arjuna's inner voice (*kṛṣṇa*)attempts to help him understand that true happiness is detaching from sensory experience and going inward to connect with the light of awareness, which requires him to act out his life duty of upholding righteousness. To reach that state, he must actively battle the parts of himself that are drawing him outward.

If we live amid a lot of hustle and bustle, tuning out that noise will be our challenge. On the other hand, if we can meditate in a quiet place, then our inner thoughts and emotions surface and distract us. This is why many ancient and modern yogins prefer to spend time in caves. Theoretically, in either environment, all distracting clamor will be rendered mute if our focus is strong enough.

A wandering heart-mind is the antithesis of yoga. Learning to focus our attention in one place helps clarify and purify our consciousness by reining in the sensory organs. The true nature of our heart-mind is transparency, which allows our inner light of awareness to shine through our being without distortion and illuminate our world with knowledge, kindness, and compassion.

THOUGHTS

Directing our focus inward rather than
outward tunes out sensory noise.

I have some control over what external stimuli I am exposed to.

I will relax my eyes, ears, tongue, nostrils, and skin as I turn my attention inward.

Exercises

The next time you are at a party, stay completely focused on your conversation, then shift your listening to other conversations. Notice how you register only sounds coming from where your attention is.

Try meditating in a noisy, busy environment. How does the external commotion affect your focus? Is tuning it out easy or difficult for you?

Try meditating in an unusually quiet environment. Notice how your internal commotion affects your focus.

45

CITTA-PRASĀDANA

Purification of the Heart-Mind

चित्तप्रसादन

Do you have the patience to wait
till your mud settles and the water is clear?
LAO-TZU

CLARITY AND PEACE OF MIND are the keys to inner and therefore outer happiness. Cultivating these qualities is given quite a bit of emphasis in the Yoga Sūtras, which mentions several methods for doing so. With a clear heart-mind, we register events accurately, communicate honestly, and live with integrity. Our inner light of awareness can shine through our transparent heart-mind and illuminate whatever we encounter, so we can perceive it truthfully.

Our social behavior, including the ethical practices called *yama-s*, can clarify our heart-mind. According to the Yoga Sūtra-s, there are also four attitudes that are to be cultivated to clarify the *citta*, correlating directly with the Buddhist *brahma-vihāra-s* or states of mind to aspire to. These are friendliness, compassion, gladness, and neutrality.

When another person is happy, be friendly toward her. Many people who are deeply unhappy in their own lives become hateful toward and envious of those who are successful or happy. Do not envy one who is happy. Cultivate contentment (*santoṣa*) by being grateful for what you have. Envy or jealousy only hurts. For example, if a colleague was promoted instead of you, congratulating her and sincerely wishing her well will purify your heart-mind. If you envy and become upset with her, you will both suffer.

When another person is suffering, being compassionate toward her sends positive, loving energy her way and helps her in her healing process. Do not avoid those who are suffering—even if they are causing you to suffer. Often, those who cause you suffering are suffering themselves. South African leader Nelson Mandela, who endured many years in prison, understood this dynamic. Instead of punishing those who made him and others suffer unjustly under apartheid, he founded the Truth and Reconciliation Commission to allow the criminals to face their victims, admit what they had done, and apologize to them. Not only did Mandela show compassion for apartheid's worst leaders, but he also provided an opportunity for them to dig deep down and express compassion toward those whose suffering they had caused.

Witnessing a virtuous act fosters a feeling of reciprocal gladness and allows us to appreciate another person. For example, a whistleblower at work speaks out about unfair or illegal activities and, in doing so, risks losing her job. This action is very courageous as this employee is risking her neck for the benefit of others. Appreciating virtuous acts such as this will encourage others to do likewise in the future.

When we encounter a person who is mean, negative, or performing illegal or unjust actions, we must step back and ask ourselves these questions: Should I get involved? What is my role here? Each individual situation will determine our level of involvement. Such involvement might include gentle caution, restraint in sharing our opinions, or complete avoidance for self-protection. It is up to you to judge the best course of action using keen discernment (*viveka*).

We may tend to shelter ourselves from anyone we consider a bad influence. Keeping good company is important for our own growth and support. Yet for us to positively affect those who need it most requires some contact. If our kindness is stronger than another's meanness, then we should be able to influence that person more than he can influence us. On the other hand, if we have not cultivated enough kindness energy, a very mean person will likely have a negative influence on us. It is important not to exclude others and to be able to interact with all sorts of people, though we also must learn who we can trust and who we should be cautious around, in order to protect our own personal progress toward inner happiness.

Arousing positive emotions as an antidote to negative emotions (*pratipakṣa-bhāvana*) purifies the heart-mind. When a negative experience inspires us to become a better person, or we put ourselves in someone else's shoes in order to understand that person's point of view, we are increasing our awareness and, thereby, clarifying our *citta*.

Turning our attention inward (by practicing *saṁyama*) refines our sensory perceptions and contributes to a clear heart-mind. The more focused we are, the better we are able to discern the truth of whatever happens around us. Our senses can be overloaded by the onslaught of information we are exposed to every day. Instead of trying to make sense of it all while immersed in it, step back into a quiet, still space and then view it from that vantage point. Watching events unfold from a quiet yet alert state of mind, we become as focused and still as a cat is just before pouncing on a mouse or nabbing a grasshopper.

The heart-mind can also be purified through *prāṇāyāma*, the fourth limb of yoga, specifically by exhaling and extending the breath, thus calming down the nervous system. To experience this type of breathwork, inhale deeply, then exhale slowly, making the exhale longer than the inhale. You'll feel a deep sense of relaxation. This stress-reducing exercise is an easy way to quiet and center yourself.

When our heart-mind is free from sorrow and filled with light, its clarification is easier. Working through our inner issues by practicing *kriyā-yoga* gradually weakens negativity and strengthens positive behavior. As we reduce our load of pain and suffering, our helpful thoughts and emotions (*vṛtti-s*) predominate, reducing the veil of ignorance (*avidyā*) and clearing the way for our inner light of awareness to illuminate our consciousness with knowledge and wisdom.

Citta-prasādana is an integral part of the gradual process of yoga. As long as we are moving ourselves in a positive direction diligently and sincerely, the residue of past experience will thin out on the lens of our heart-mind, and our ever-present light of knowledge can be experienced within.

THOUGHTS

Purification and clarification of my heart-mind
field are central to the practice of yoga.

I endeavor to remove negativity from my mind so
the inner light of awareness can shine through.

I will cultivate an attitude of friendliness, compassion, and
joy while maintaining healthy and appropriate boundaries.

EXERCISES

At work, when a colleague who may be vying for a similar promotion as you are receives a pat on the back for an excellent project, be happy for him. Always encourage others to succeed. May the best win!

At a sporting event, when the team playing against the team you are cheering for makes an amazing play that wins the game, swallow your pride and give them credit for a game well played.

The next time you witness a crime or hurtful action, think carefully before deciding on a course of action.

46

DHĀRAṆĀ

Choosing a Focus

धारणा

Except for the point, the still point,
There would be no dance, and there is only the dance.
T. S. ELIOT, "Burnt Norton," *Four Quartets*

THE FIRST STEP TO UNDERSTANDING something is choosing to engage it and attempting to connect with it. Keen discernment (*viveka*) is necessary for choosing carefully and wisely, since the object chosen will influence our consciousness as we spend time deliberately focusing on it. With ongoing effort and patience, we will eventually be able to comprehend its essence deeply.

Dhāraṇā, which is the sixth of the eight limbs of yoga (*aṣṭāṅga*), is the initial stage of turning inward, a three-stage process called *saṁyama*. *Dhāraṇā* is defined as "keeping the attention on a single place." At this stage, one proactively chooses an object to focus on. The object can be an external physical thing, an abstract idea, or (more traditionally) an internal aspect of ourselves.

Examples of external objects include a flame, an image, or even an idol. We should like the object, but not be attached to it in any way. If there is any resistance to it, or if it brings up negative or distracting thoughts, then something else should be selected. The object should have the qualities of *sattva.* For example, let's say you choose an image of Jesus. After meditating on that particular image, you realize that it resembles an acquaintance you do not care for. If the idea of Jesus as sacred gets corrupted by your memory of this other person, it is time to either find a different image of Jesus or choose an entirely different object of focus.

Alternatively, choosing a person who we want to understand better can greatly benefit our relationship with him. For example, a teacher can focus on his students' well-being and development, or a close friend may spend time pondering a difficult issue of yours to help us make a better decision about how to resolve it. Contemplative and optimistic attention concentrated on any person or situation will energetically benefit all parties.

Ideas can also be a place of focus. If we wish to understand an abstract concept more fully, then quiet contemplation on it can open it up and allow us to access on a very deep level what the concept is all about. Inventors and scientists consciously ruminate so often that when they stop, their unconscious continues the contemplation, often resulting in brilliant ideas.

Inner objects of focus may include a *cakra,* mantra, the breath, or even the divine within us. A traditional and common place of focus is the heart area/*cakra,* regarded as the center of our being. It is said in the Katha Upaniṣad that a flame the size of a thumb burns continuously in the heart, like a pilot light of life. This glow represents the warm, inner splendor of pure awareness.

Dhāraṇā alone can be intermittent—attention drifting away, then back again. When it becomes continuous, then we have reached the second stage of *saṁyama,* which is called *dhyāna.* In *dhāraṇā,* we are aware of our surroundings, but they do not distract our focus very much. In *dhyāna*, peripheral commotion does not cause any distraction.

The regulation of our breath (*prāṇāyāma*) prepares the heart-mind for *dhāraṇā*. This stage of the eight limbs of yoga (*aṣṭāṅga*) is when we rein in our wandering and distracted attention. Choose something to focus on, place your attention there, and be as still as possible. With detached awareness (*vairāgya*), we can begin to perceive the object objectively, setting aside our baggage, and allowing our field of consciousness to fully experience its true essence.

THOUGHTS

The first step to directing the attention
inward is choosing an object of focus.

I can carefully select an object that does
not disturb my heart-mind.

I will focus my attention on this object of
focus and try to keep it there.

EXERCISES

Choose a person whom you would like to understand better. Sit quietly and probe into why this person behaves the way she does. Is there a way to accept this person for who she is and not react when conflict arises between the two of you?

Sit quietly and bring your attention to your breath.
Feel yourself relaxing with each inhalation and
exhalation. Notice any irregularities in the breath
and how they affect your consciousness.

Sit quietly and focus on the divine within
you, seated in the area of your heart.

47

DHYĀNA

Continuous Focus

ध्यान

Your vision will become clear only when you look into your heart. Who looks outside, dreams. Who looks inside, awakens.

CARL JUNG

THE SECOND STEP TO UNDERSTANDING something or someone happens naturally as your concentration lasts longer and the distractions within and without lessen. This one-pointedness awakens us to our inner peace and brings us one step closer to complete absorption (*samādhi*). With *dhyāna*, the heart-mind begins to clarify (*citta-prasādana*), and the detrimental thoughts and emotions (*kliṣṭa-vṛtti-s*) fade away.

Dhyāna is the seventh limb of yoga and the middle stage of turning inward (*saṁyama*). *Dhyāna* is continuous *dhāraṇā*, attention so focused that peripheral noise does not interfere with our concentration. *Dhāraṇā* is focusing on a single object, but thoughts about the object vary. *Dhyāna* occurs when only a single idea is present in the heart-mind. As an archer concentrates only on the bull's eye and nothing else, we focus only on our chosen object. In *dhyāna*, only one thought about the object exists. *Dhāraṇā* is like water dripping intermittently on a single spot; *dhyāna* is like honey flowing continuously over the spot.

An unfocused heart-mind is, by definition, fragmented and distracted. As our attention drifts from one thing to another quickly, our nervous system amps up, affecting our breath and creating stress on our body. Performing too many tasks at once in a limited amount of time is a recipe for disquietude and stress. If we do this day in and day out, we move toward a consciousness taken up entirely by a multitude of thoughts and emotions, and further and further away from our true nature.

Dhyāna can be practiced wherever full concentration is helpful. For example, at the end of an *āsana* practice, it is helpful to sit quietly in order to transition from the practice to the next activity in your day. Even while doing a posture, if you are fully focused on your body or breath, then you are practicing *dhyāna*. Each time your attention strays to a fellow classmate or the teacher, you revert back to *dhāraṇā*. Early in the morning, especially before sunrise, is considered the best time to meditate, since very little is going on. Whenever we turn our attention inward, we usually shift among the three inner limbs of yoga (*dhāraṇā*, *dhyāna*, and *samādhi*).

Dhyāna can help us overcome detrimental thoughts and emotions (*kliṣṭa-vṛtti-s*) that are the result of deeper mental-emotional triggers (*kleśa-s*). During *dhyāna*, there is room for only one *vṛtti* in the heart-mind, the current and continuous thought directed toward the focal point. Because of this, *dhyāna* blocks out the afflictive thoughts and emotions, allowing our heart-mind to absorb only the positive energy of the chosen object.

For example, as we concentrate on understanding others, we see their positive and negative aspects as nothing more than an accumulation of their past experience. The more time we spend seeing their outer appearance as a temporary shell covering up their true nature, the closer we are to the last stage of turning inward (*samādhi*). If our chosen object is our heart, then we realize the same holds true for ourselves.

The clarification and stabilization of the heart-mind (*citta-prasādana*) can result from *dhyāna* as well. The more the attention is focused, the fewer distractions occur, and the more the heart-mind becomes serene and composed. Eventually, as our heart-mind becomes immersed in the pure waters of meditation, it will no longer produce any negative behavioral patterns (*saṁskāra-s*), paving the way for us to become a kinder and more compassionate presence.

As we become transfixed on our chosen object, we bolster our inner orientation and let go of outer distractions, and the final limb of yoga (*samādhi*) inches closer and closer. *Dhyāna* is the centerpiece of turning inward and is necessary for connecting with our divine inner light of awareness.

THOUGHTS

As the heart-mind concentrates on its chosen object,
peripheral distractions gradually fade away.

I can maintain my focus continuously,
disregarding all other activity.

I will continue to progress toward complete
understanding of my chosen object.

EXERCISES

Choose a person to focus on, and set aside time each day to meditate on that person in order to gradually understand who she or he is and, if you have issues with that person, when and why he or she pushes your buttons.

The next time you are interacting one-on-one with a person while others are present, see if you can keep your attention on the person you are talking with instead of listening in on other nearby conversations.

While you are meditating, are you seeking something? See if you can practice patience and let go of results, allowing your heart-mind to settle naturally on your chosen object and being in no hurry to reach any particular state. Just *be* with the object.

48

SAMĀDHI

Complete Attention

समाधि

The birds have vanished into the sky
and now the last cloud drains away.
We sit together, the mountain and me,
until only the mountain remains.
LI PO, translated from the Chinese by Sam Hamill

WHEN WE ARE SO COMPLETELY focused that our own sense of individuality vanishes, then our heart-mind field of consciousness (*citta*) reflects only the object of focus and nothing else. Our attention is so riveted and unswerving that external sensory input is totally turned off (*pratyāharā*). We are in a zone, having let go of the outer world, and now experience a feeling of unity.

Samādhi is the eighth and final limb of *aṣṭāṅga-yoga* and is functionally identical to yoga as the state of *nirodha*. At this stage, there is no perception of a subject separate from its object. Both seem to be one entity, uniting in the heart-mind's eye even though in physical reality the practitioner is still different from the object. Yoga is often defined as "union" in this sense. In *samādhi*, the ego takes a vacation; it is removed from the equation since it can function only when the object can be distinguished from the subject.

Since the heart-mind needs a prop to enable it to move toward stillness, it relies on an object. During this final limb of yoga, the object of focus is still present even though we cannot distinguish it as separate from our heart-mind. Beyond this state, when our *citta* does not even reflect the object and becomes transparent, is the ultimate goal of full connection with our divine inner light of awareness (*puruṣa*).

Samādhi can be experienced in everyday life. Anytime we get lost in something and our consciousness is completely absorbed in it, we are experiencing a type of *samādhi*. Full participation in an activity, when we are so involved in it that nothing else exists except what we are focused on doing, can be *samādhi*. A hypnotic trance is another example. Intoxication and addiction can be considered harmful types of *samādhi-s*. The *samādhi* defined by Patañjali as the final stage of *saṁyama* is conscious and has the qualities of *sattva*.

One way of looking at *samādhi* is as a sequence of steps toward complete mastery of an object—knowing everything about the object inside and out. These steps progress from a superficial to a deep level of understanding.

1. The most superficial stage is when our heart-mind attempts to understand the object by means of our intellect alone, through reasoning, logic, inference, or conjecture. Here, objects are identified by words, and each word may be interpreted differently among different people. What the object is or is not is debatable, and our opinions on it are influenced by our mental-emotional afflictions (*kleśa-s*). For example, let's say we are learning to play a musical instrument. At this stage, we can play notes from the sheet

music or by ear, basic chord progressions, and key changes. We have a good, basic, yet superficial understanding and technique. We may have a strong attachment to playing the instrument (*rāga*) or an intense aversion (*dveṣa*) because we are forced into taking lessons.

2. The second stage is a subtler, deeper attempt of the mind to understand an object, with more careful examination and reflection. We now use keen, refined discernment and reflection to get to a more accurate and truthful evaluation of the object. The qualities of the object are no longer debatable, nor are they influenced by our mental-emotional afflictions (*kleśa-s.*) Irrational ideas that stun the mind, like those of a Zen koan, occur at this level. To continue our example, we now understand how tempo and volume affect the feeling of the music we are playing.

3. The joy and satisfaction of fully understanding something occurs in the third stage. The knowledge temporarily becomes part of us, and we really enjoy being able to experience it. We can now play the musical piece by heart.

4. When the knowledge becomes completely internalized, becomes part of our identity, then the object is said to have merged with us, the subject. This complete mastery allows us the freedom to experiment with new, unknown ideas. Using our example, we can now play a piece perfectly, without having to think about it, yet with awareness of our surroundings. We do not even need to look at our fingers or hand.

According to the *sūtra-s*, one who has enough faith in the divine (*īśvara-praṇidhāna*), who truly sees the divine light inside all beings, can bypass the normal stages of development and reach the final state of *samādhi* directly. Reaching *samādhi* this way is considered very rare.

Most practitioners begin with faith in their own ability to move ahead and inward. Faith provides the determination, enthusiasm, and energy that supports a clear memory and leads to the deep insight of *samādhi*. Without faith, we succumb to doubt, which, like fire, consumes everything in its path.

There is no rush. Cultivating a clear heart-mind field requires time, patience, and practice. The level (mild, medium, or ardent) and frequency of our practice creates momentum that accelerates our progress. As long as we practice regularly and with sincere effort, gradual inner progress will happen, and it will manifest as more happiness, contentment, and joy.

THOUGHTS

When the heart-mind becomes transparent,
it perfectly reflects what it perceives.

By focusing so completely on one object, my heart-mind
perceives no difference between it and me.

I will recognize the light of awareness in every
sentient being and see others as part of myself.

Exercises

Can you remember anytime in the past when you found yourself "in the zone," whether it was during meditation, physical activity, or something else? What did it feel like, and how long did the feeling last?

Choose an activity and see if you can focus so intently on it that nothing else seems to exist.

Sit quietly in a pain-free position (there is nothing wrong with using a chair) and bring your attention to the inner light of awareness seated near your heart center. Meditate without moving until you experience a feeling of oneness with the inner light of awareness.

49

SAṀYAMA

Focusing Inward

संयम

Only a one-pointed mind, turned inward,
succeeds in Self-inquiry.
RAMANA MAHARSHI

THE PROCESS OF TURNING OUR attention away from outer objects and toward our inner Self occurs in stages and is the culmination of our journey through the eight limbs of yoga (*aṣṭāṅga*). The previous limbs are preparation for *saṁyama*, which itself can mean meditation.

Saṁyama is the practice of the final three "inner" limbs of yoga, all focused on a single place or object. At this point, due to *prāṇāyāma*, the breath should be stable and without obstruction or irregularity. As our heart-mind turns inward and progresses from one stage of *saṁyama* to the next, outer sensory stimuli fade away (*pratyāhāra*) naturally and completely.

According to the Yoga Sūtras, the application of *saṁyama* occurs in three stages. As we sit quietly for meditation, we will most likely move back and forth among them, eventually spending less time in the first stage and more time in the last.

Most practitioners need to progress step-by-step, gradually refining their heart-mind from outer, coarser thoughts toward inner, subtler thoughts.

Saṁyama begins with choosing an object or location and attempting to focus on that (*dhāraṇā*). At this point, we are developing our ability to focus, and our attention on the object is intermittent, like water dripping from a faucet. When we are able to focus our attention continuously, like water flowing in an unbroken stream, then *dhyāna* is occurring. Finally, when our attention is complete and there is no perceivable difference between ourselves and the object, *samādhi* is experienced. The object of focus is empty of independent existence and no longer appears to be a separate entity from ourselves. We seem to be the water.

Saṁyama can also be applied to an outer object for the purpose of understanding it better. For example, you have been in an on-and-off relationship for a few years. You are meeting other people that you are attracted to. Should you commit to working through the issues of the relationship, or should you just end it and move on, hoping a better one will come along? Practicing *saṁyama* on this decision may shed enough light on it that you can finally leave your frustrating state of limbo.

From mastery of *saṁyama* comes the light of deep insight. Understanding of the object of focus is complete from the inside out and extends to all levels (gross to subtle). From that penetrating insight arise extraordinary abilities. According to Patañjali, these supernatural powers are side effects that are to be ignored or only noticed, never abused or demonstrated, and that are obstacles to moving closer to permanent oneness (*kaivalya*).

These extraordinary abilities can also be developed in other ways. Some people are born with supernormal powers, such as clairvoyance or extrasensory perception (ESP). The external and/or internal application of concentrated medicinal concoctions is said to allow one to achieve these special abilities as well. So can chanting a mantra or practicing intense *tapas*. *Samādhi* is considered the best way to develop these abilities, because they are side effects of a pure and virtuous discipline, not a deliberate attempt to gain power.

Saṁyama is interiorizing the object of focus, ultimately making it appear as if it *is* the *citta*. As we progress through the phases, we cultivate an inner orientation by becoming less interested in outer pursuits. Turning our attention inward is easier after practicing the previous limbs of yoga, which prepare us for this final journey toward our true nature.

THOUGHTS

The inner limbs of yoga draw me toward the
pure, inner light that is my true nature.

I can remain focused and attentive no matter
what extraordinary abilities develop.

I will seek simplicity and peace, not power or prestige.

EXERCISES

Have you ever witnessed or personally experienced
supernormal powers? Imagine having such powers
yourself, and see what this brings up in your heart-mind.

Sit in a comfortable position with a vertical spine. Quietly contemplate a chosen outer object, like a decision that needs to be made or a person you are having difficulty with. How can you more fully understand the object? Probe deeper and deeper until more knowledge about it is revealed. How does this knowledge change your view of the object?

Meditate inwardly on a chosen inner object. Notice every physical distraction and try to rectify it. Whenever you realize that your attention has drifted, bring it back to your object. Pretend the object is inside of your consciousness, not outside.

50

PRATIPRASAVA

Returning to the Source

प्रतिप्रसव

It is by going down into the abyss that we recover the treasures of life. Where you stumble, there lies your treasure.
JOSEPH CAMPBELL

UNDERSTANDING OUR PAST CAN REVEAL why we act the way we do now, and our actions now will affect how we behave in the future. We are the result of our experiences. Our negative thoughts, feelings, and reactions today can give us clues with which to begin an investigation into our past.

Yoga is partly about getting to know who we are inside and why we act the way we do. Whenever we react automatically to a stimulus, instead of stepping back and acting consciously, we allow our deep triggers (*kleśa-s*), habitual patterns (*saṁskāra-s*), and mental commotion (*vṛtti-s*) to determine our reaction. To prevent this, we can learn from the suffering our reaction causes (*duḥkha*), trace our reaction back to its source (*pratiprasava*), and discover what caused it. What happened in my past that made me act this way? How can I improve myself so that I act in a way I am proud of and feel good about?

Just as the only way to truly eliminate disease is to remove its cause, so the only way to get rid of negative and harmful reactions is to destroy their seeds within us: either mental-emotional afflictions (*kleśa-s*) or strong habitual patterns (*saṁskāra-s*). *Kleśa-s* are weakened by practicing *kriyā-yoga* and dissolved by *pratiprasava*. Negative *saṁskāra-s* fade away when other positive *saṁskāra-s* become strong enough to supersede them.

If we notice when a *kleśa* is manifesting in a subtle form and view it as a warning sign or symptom of something deeper, we can nip it in the bud before it controls our actions. For example, let's say you composed a song that became a big hit. All of a sudden, you are famous, and many people are throwing their attention your way. If you notice yourself (*svādhyāya*) beginning to feel better than others (*asmitā-kleśa*), and understand where your feeling of superiority came from, there is an opportunity to pass the credit through your heart-mind to something higher than yourself (*īśvara*) by practicing *īśvara-praṇidhāna*. This stops the rising *asmitā-kleśa* by turning it around and sending it back to dormancy (*pratiprasava*). If you are vigilant enough, you can save yourself from conceit. Otherwise, as the ego accepts and holds on to all that attention, *asmitā-kleśa* grows inside your heart-mind like a noxious weed and will be much more difficult to remove.

Reflecting on our *kleśa-s* and *saṁskāra-s* even when they are not active allows us to prepare ourselves for their inevitable arousal. For example, whenever you are in the presence of pastries or donuts, you cannot help eating some, even though you are trying to lose weight. If you promise yourself that the next time they are available, you will think of them as poison to your system, then maybe when the temptation arises again you will be able to nip it in the bud and restrain yourself from eating those fatty foods.

Pratiprasava is a powerful exercise and is necessary to end the *kleśa-s* and any remaining negative or positive *saṁskāra-s,* the final step before *kaivalya.* As our heart-mind clears and we are able to remember past events that left a strong imprint in our consciousness, our current behavior might start to make more sense. Replacing longstanding habitual patterns with new ones requires diligence, focus, and persistence over a long period of time (*abhyāsa*). Eventually, our heart and mind become purified and able to enjoy the sweet taste of our inner light of awareness.

THOUGHTS

Discovering where a detrimental thought pattern originally came from can help end it.

When I gain insight into the way I think and act habitually, I truly understand myself better.

I will find out what past impressions cause me to react unconsciously and take steps to resolve them.

EXERCISES

The next time you are tempted by cigarettes, sweets, or some other substance that creates a bad reaction in your system, watch your thoughts and see what you tell yourself about the substance. You can also step back and observe your thoughts and self-talk when experiencing a particular emotional state, to see what beliefs underlie your emotion.

Sit quietly and meditate on your past, especially those events or actions that may have left a deep impression in your psyche. Write them down, and note what current behaviors might be the results of them.

Think about what situations cause you to react to an immediate family member. Then sit down with that family member or another immediate kin and ask him or her where it comes from. You can do this with a very old friend as well.

51

KAIVALYA

Permanent Oneness

कैवल्य

This little light of mine, I'm gonna let it shine.
HARRY DIXON LOES, from THIS LITTLE LIGHT OF MINE

THE CULMINATION OF YOGA PRACTICE occurs when our heart-mind is completely pure and our "buttons" are gone. This state of equanimity is a lofty goal that few attain. Yet even in the very likely event that this goal is never reached, engaging in the practices of yoga will improve life immensely. It's more about the means than the end, the journey rather than the goal. Why not aim high and enjoy the benefits of moving toward the goal?

Kaivalya literally means "aloneness" and is the final state of emancipation, where we are not affected by any conditioning in our heart-mind whatsoever. The inner light of awareness shines right through our consciousness to illuminate the world around us, turning any action into a selfless, compassionate offering to that awareness. *Kaivalya* cannot be understood with words; it requires direct experience. During the process of self-refinement, the effect of yoga practice, glimpses of our inner light of awareness occur more and more often as our heart-mind becomes clarified.

Kaivalya can be interpreted in many different ways, using many different words, none of which can do justice to the actual experience. Some English words and phrases that may reflect some characteristics of *kaivalya* are *permanent oneness, quiet simplicity, conscious isolation, emancipation, freedom, liberation,* and *enlightenment.*.

As our heart-mind clears, it returns back to its true nature of *sattva,* exhibiting all positive qualities, such as virtue, nonviolence, kindness, and compassion. As wonderful as this sounds, it is not quite the end. Even the aforementioned qualities can bind us to the outer world. If our ego thinks, "I am now filled with *sattva,*" then we might regard ourselves as better than those whose heart-minds are not there yet. It is crucial to distinguish between a *sattvic* heart-mind and the inner light of awareness that is devoid of any qualities at all.

Once the distinction is made between a *sattvic citta* and the *puruṣa,* a sequence of steps occurs, leading us to *kaivalya.* Our sense of self ceases. All *karma* and *kleśa-s* end. Clear, untainted access to all knowledge (*īśvara*) occurs. Perception of time stops, since time exists only in the manifest world (*dṛśya*). A continuous, unbroken *viveka* is present, and we are fully content and not interested in moving forward anymore. Trying and seeking come to an end, and full relaxation of the heart-mind ensues. The power of pure awareness rests in its own nature.

There have been accounts of people considered to be enlightened. It is important to distinguish between a person who teaches about spirituality and one who has attained *kaivalya.* Many teachers, well versed in the ancient scriptures, can transfix an audience with their knowledge and charisma—yet behind the scenes they act unethically. A truly enlightened being will have no interest in power, money, or fame. With a healthy ego, he or she will treat all others equally and will never abuse the sacred relationship with his or her followers. Sitting in the presence of this person calms and quiets us, and asking questions seems pointless. She or he is like a clear mirror that shows us exactly who we are.

There are many paths to the same goal. The path of the Yoga Sūtras, which can be considered scientific and/or religious, is only one. Every religion has its own ways of connecting with the divine and its own names for it, just as each culture has its own customs, rituals, and view of the world. Accepting other ways of living and allowing other people to pursue their own paths enables freedom of expression and promotes tolerance and peace. No religion or philosophy has exclusive access to that which is independent of all of them. Such thinking has caused significant conflict and violence throughout the course of history.

Our society has become quite complex. The path of yoga moves us toward simplicity and the ordinary. As our heart-mind quiets down and focuses on one thing, we cultivate an inner orientation that develops contentment and spiritual maturity. Our interactions with others improve as friendliness and compassion grow. Life becomes easier and simpler as our attention is disentangled from the outer world. As we unravel the layers of our conditioning, we experience more and more of the soft, warm, unassuming glow that is our true essence. *Kaivalya* is the freedom to simply be.

THOUGHTS

I look forward to spending time alone with myself.

I strive for a quiet, content heart-mind
that enjoys moments of solitude.

Realizing that everything changes over time gives me a sense of nonattachment and freedom from the external world.

EXERCISES

Sit quietly and contemplate the purpose of seeking the extraordinary. Is it your ego that seeks this? How will seeking the extraordinary help you be content? See if you can be happy with only yourself and nothing else.

Think about what you are seeking. If it is on the outside, are you attached to it? Maybe it is a spiritual teacher who directs you inward. If so, when this teacher dies, will you mourn his outer form or continue your journey inward, meeting the teacher's essence any time you wish?

Are you comfortable being alone? If not, why?

EPILOGUE

INTERPRETATIONS OF THE YOGA SŪTRAS can vary and have been debated for thousands of years. A Hindu *swāmī* will more likely teach according to the words written by the generally accepted commentators, most notably Veda Vyāsa. An American New Age writer may publish a looser, more poetic translation that appeals to a different audience. For centuries, commentaries upon commentaries have been written on the Yoga Sūtras, agreeing and disagreeing in various ways. Practically speaking, it is of paramount importance to express what the author Patañjali is saying in a way that retains much of the traditional meaning, yet is understandable to everyone and useful when applied to everyday living.

Patañjali made sure his presentation was not limited to geography, culture, religion, or even time period. The philosophy of yoga so eloquently written in these *sūtra-s* is truly universal and nonsectarian. Principles such as nonviolence, truthfulness, and nonstealing are common among many religions and philosophies of the world. There is only one word in this text that can be translated as "lord," and that is *īśvara*, which can be interpreted simply as something greater than ourselves.

The golden rule, "Do unto others as you would have them do unto you," is another way of expressing the law of *karma* and the inner meaning of *namaste*, or "I bow to the divine within you." A focus on self-development and clarification of the heart-mind makes the application and pursuit of yoga good for all people and for society as a whole.

The worldview of ancient India, and, therefore, of yoga, is fundamentally different than ours. We have separated ourselves from nature and attached ourselves to material possessions, most of which are man-made syntheses of elements and chemicals extracted from nature herself. Ours is a world focused on outer pursuits and wealth, often demanding hard evidence before believing something is true. People with an ambition to acquire external possessions are rewarded, while a quieter, more contemplative person is considered boring and unappealing to be around.

Yoga is concerned primarily with turning our attention inward in order to understand who we are. Intellectual knowledge is considered a bridge to the goal, not the goal in itself. Wisdom comes from direct experience with both outer events and inner contemplation. Stillness is priceless, carrying much more value than the temporary pleasures and pains of the outside world. The divine is always inside and part of us, not outside looking down on us. All outer things are impermanent, unconscious entities, while our inner light of awareness is permanent and conscious.

This difference in worldview may be what attracts us to yoga. We are longing to connect to our inner being, longing to experience that simple inner happiness that does not depend on outer, changing circumstances. Cultivating an inner orientation and discovering who we really are will energetically transform our attitudes and encourage kindness and compassion.

PERMISSIONS AND CREDITS

Chapter 4: "All creeping things..." from the book *Dumpling Field: Haiku of Issa* translated by Lucien Stryk with the assistance of Noboru Fujiwara. Reprinted with the permission of Swallow Press/Ohio University Press, Athens, Ohio (ohioswallow.com).

Chapter 12: "The dark thought..." from "The Guest House" from *The Essential Rumi*, HarperCollins, 1995, by permission of translator Coleman Barks.

Chapter 48: "The birds have vanished..." from "Zazen on Ching-t'ing Mountain" from *Crossing the Yellow River: Three Hundred Poems from the Chinese*, BOA Editions, 2000, by permission of the translator, Sam Hamill.

Translations of Sanskrit verses from the Bhagavad Gītā, Yoga Sūtras, and Śrī Guru Strotram by Nicolai Bachman.

FOR FURTHER STUDY

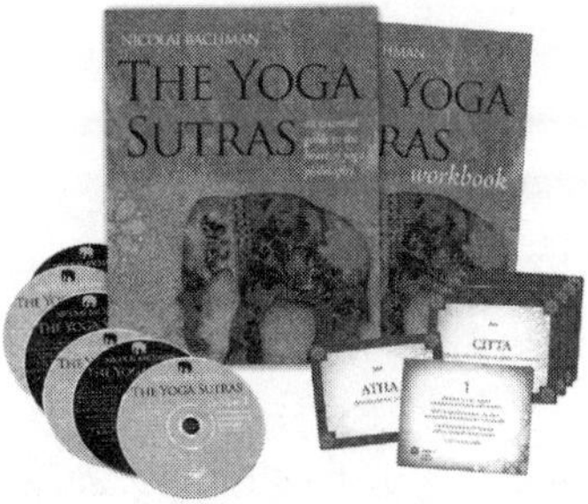

THE YOGA SUTRAS
An Essential Guide to the Heart of Yoga Philosophy
Boulder, CO: Sounds True, 2010

Aligned with *The Path of the Yoga Sutras: A Practical Guide to the Core of Yoga*, this is a comprehensive home-study course for those who want to go deeper into the sūtras in terms of Sanskrit, chanting, and processes of yoga. The same core yoga principles are discussed, but in a much more comprehensive manner. Whether you're a seasoned teacher or a student looking to go deeper with your practice, this essential course offers a treasury of teachings to further your study of yoga. Each of the fifty-one important concepts has an inspirational card, a full commentary in the book, and an audio track on one of the CDs. This set includes:

- A 336-page letter-size workbook with
  - a concise history of yoga and the sūtras
  - in-depth explanation of all fifty-one key themes
  - a full word-by-word translation of all 195 sūtras, including the original Sanskrit script and transliteration for every sūtra

- thirteen full-color diagrams, flow charts, and tables illustrating key processes of yoga
- an outline of the sūtras in translation only, grouped to see a bird's eye view of the meaning of all the sūtras
- a list of sūtras in order of their first word, to find a sūtra easily if you know its first few syllables
- an appendix showing the Yoga Sutras in their original Sanskrit script alone
- an appendix in large typeface for chanting the sūtras along with the seventh CD
- other appendices on the three *gunas* (*sattva, rajas,* and *tamas*), the powers from chapter 3, and the six philosophical systems from India, of which yoga is one
- a complete glossary of Sanskrit terms for quick reference

• Six CDs full of insights to further your learning about the fifty-one essential principles

• A seventh CD for learning to chant the complete text, following along with a chanting section in the workbook

• Fifty-one study cards to encourage reflection of each concept and inspire action

FURTHER RESOURCES

Yoga Sutras Interpretations

Bouanchaud, Bernard. *The Essence of Yoga; Reflections on the Yoga Sutras of Patañjali.* Portland, Oregon: Rudra Press, 1997. (RT, ET, DEF). Refined and practical interpretation. One sūtra per page with reflections to contemplate on each sūtra. Full index of terms in the back.

Bryant, Edwin. *The Yoga Sūtras of Patañjali.* New York, New York: North Point Press, 2009. (SS, RT, ET, VV, DEF). Excellent traditional and academic interpretation. He includes relevant ideas from every major commentator, with copious endnotes and bibliography.

Desikachar, T.K.V. *The Heart of Yoga.* Rochester, Vermont: Inner Traditions International, 1995. (SS, RT, ET). Loose yet practical interpretation with brief commentary. Book includes much more than the sūtras.

Hariharananda Aranya, Swami. *Yoga Philosophy of Patañjali.* Albany: State University of New York Press, 1983. (SS, ET, VV, COM). The most comprehensive, with long commentaries on the sūtra and on Vyasa's commentary. A very traditional interpretation.

Hartranft, Chip. *The Yoga-Sūtra of Patañjali*. Boston, Massachusetts: Shambhala Publications, Inc., 2003. arlingtoncenter.org (ET, COM). Smooth and clear explanation in English, with a slightly Buddhist leaning.

Houston, Vyaas. *The Yoga Sūtra Workbook: The Certainty of Freedom*. Warwick, New York: American Sanskrit Institute, 1995. americansanskrit.com (SS, RT, ET, DEF, GR). Translation is literal with no commentary. One sūtra per letter-size page with plenty of room for notes. Spiral-bound.

Iyengar, B.K.S. *Light on the Yoga Sūtras of Patañjali*. San Francisco, California: Aquarian/Thorsons (Harper Collins), 1993. (SS, RT, ET, DEF, COM). Excellent reference, includes many tables, great indices in the back. A very traditional interpretation.

SS = Sanskrit Script
RT = Romanized Transliteration
ET = English Translation
VV = Veda Vyaas's commentary on the Yoga Sutras
DEF = Definitions of each individual word
GR = Grammatical endings shown

INDEX

A

abhiniveśa (fear of death), 106, **129–131**

abhyāsa (diligent, focused practice), **29–32,** 34, 36, 47, 77, 102, 110, 247
  necessity of, 30–31, 35
  supported by *viveka*, 27

action. See *karma*

addiction, 34, 52, 120, 129, 236

afflictions, mental-emotional. See *kleśa-s*

ahiṁsā (nonviolence and compassion), 140, **143–147,** 153, 176, 191
  satya and, 149–150

anger, 67, 123, 124, 143, 144, 166

antarāya-s (obstacles that distract), 31, 45, 91, **99–103,** 202, 209, 212

anxiety, 34, 83, 176, 201

aparigraha (nonhoarding), 140, **161–164**

apathy, 31, 99, 100, 209

Aristotle, 149

Arjuna, 51, 218–219

āsana (refinement of the body), **207–210**
  importance of, 208
  as third limb of yoga, 1–2, 136

asmitā (distorted sense of self), 72, **113–117,** 246

aṣṭāṅga (eight limbs of yoga), 40, **135–137**

asteya (not taking from others), 140, **153–156**

atha (readiness and commitment), **7–10**

ātman, 17. See *puruṣa* (pure inner light of awareness)

attachment, xx, 21, 27, 32, 51, 108, 129, 131, 141, 158, 163, 202, 205, 209, 217, 237
  clinging to past pleasure (*rāga*), 119–120, 122
  nonattachment, 252. See also
    vairāgya

attention. See also focus, *samādhi*
  breath (*prāṇāyāma*) and, 218
  complete (*samādhi*), 235–239
  turning inward, 73, 241–244, 254

aversion. See *dveṣa*

avidyā (lack of awareness), 72, 83, 105, 106, **109–112,** 114, 166, 203, 209, 224
removing, 22–23, 110–111

awareness, xvi, xvii, 41, 51, 72, 76, 125, 192, 195, 197, 209, 223, 229, 237

Ayurveda, 1, 157, 176, 209

B

beginner's mind, 8

Bhagavad-Gītā, 17, 51, 91, 197, 218–219

brahmacarya (conservation of vital energy), 140, **157–159,** 191

breath/breathing, xvii, 2, 3, 17, 19, 31, 58, 99, 102, 147, 158, 172, 190, 209, 224, 228, 230, 232. See also *prāṇā; prāṇāyāma*

Buddha, 1, 33

C

cakra, 212, 228

Campbell, Joseph, 99, 245

carelessness, 99, 100, 101

cause and effect, 144. See *karma*

change, xv, xx, 7, 8, 15, 19, 34, 52, 59, 115, 123, 130, 162, 171, 178. See also *dṛśya; kriyā-yoga; pariṇāma; tapas*
suffering and, 66–67

chi, 211

citta (heart-mind field of consciousness), **11–15,** 22, 65, 72, 88, 92, 96, 99, 107, 109, 111, 179, 195, 235, 236, 243. See also *citta-prasādana*
positive, uplifting company/focus and, 13, 50, 223
sattvic citta, 250
silencing (*yoga as nirodha*), 39, 40

citta-prasādana (purification of the heart-mind), 12, 13, 19, 77, 83, 85, 96, 186, 213, **221–225,** 231, 233. See also *citta*

cleanliness. See *śauca*

commitment. See *atha*

committed effort. See *abhyāsa*

company, good and bad, 13, 27, 50, 114, 223

compassion, 3, 17, 18, 19, 40, 49, 76, 81, 124, 151, 167, 219, 221, 222, 224, 233, 249, 250, 251, 254. See also *ahiṁsā*

Confucius, 185

consciousness, heart-mind field of. See *citta*

conservation of vital energy. See *brahmacarya*

contentment. See *santoṣa*

cravings, 33, 159

creation, 43, 45. See also *Om*

D

darkness. See *avidyā*

darśana, 23

daydreams, 37, 88, 90

death, 50, 58, 79, 162, 177, 211. See also *abhiniveśa*

delusion, 40, 67, 72, 76, 84, 88, 101, 113, 115, 144, 166

desires, 67, 89, 124, 140, 144, 155. See also *rāga; vairāgya*

directing inward, 34–36
sexual, 158–159

dhāraṇā (choosing a focus), **227–230**
dhyāna and, 231–232
as limb of yoga, 136, 227, 229
as part of *saṁyama* (focusing inward), 227, 242

dhyāna (continuous focus), 77, 107, 172, 228, 229, **231–234,** 242
as limb of yoga, 136, 231

discernment/discrimination. See *viveka*

disease, 31, 45, 53, 87, 99–100, 107, 209, 212, 246

distractions, xvi, 3, 13, 30, 32, 45, 88, 92, 110, 157, 158, 177, 191, 201, 208, 228, 229, 244. See also *antarāya-s; dhyāna; pratyāhāra; vṛtti-s; yoga as nirodha*

"do unto others" rule, 49, 253

Dogen, Eihei, 195

doubt/self-doubt, 31, 45, 99, 100, 114, 202, 238

dreams, xvi, 90, 93, 23. See also *daydreams*
dream sleep, 91–92

dṛśya (ever-changing Mother Nature), **21–24,** 59, 71, 73, 190, 250

duḥkha, 26, 60, **65–69,** 72, 110, 119, 166, 180, 190, 191, 245

dveṣa (clinging to past suffering), 35, 106, 120, **123–127,** 130, 176, 196, 237

E

ego/egotism, 3, 12, 19, 27, 40, 44, 72, 76, 84, 108, 129, 145, 146, 161–163, 176, 201, 202–203, 205, 236, 246, 250, 251, 252. See also *asmitā*

eight limbs of yoga, 2, 14, 139, 145. See also *aṣṭāṅga*

Einstein, Albert, 139, 153

emotions, xiv, xvi, 8, 11, 13, 17, 19, 24, 30, 39, 42, 53, 58, 68, 92–93, 107, 111, 119–121, 130, 165, 167, 176, 177, 181, 190, 196, 202, 211, 219, 223, 231, 232, 248. See also *asmitā; dveṣa; kleśa-s; kliṣṭa-vṛtti-s; rāga; vṛtti-s; yoga as nirodha*

energy, conservation of vital. See *brahmacarya*

enlightenment. See *kaivalya*

envy, 67, 154, 156, 222

ESP, 242

ethical practices. See *yama-s*

evaluation, correct. See *pramāṇa*

F

faith. See *īśvara-praṇidhāna*

false identification of seer with seen. See *saṁyoga*

father, 22, 97

fatigue, 99, 101

fear, 34, 97, 105, 108, 110, 112, 114, 119, 123, 125, 129–130, 202. See also *abhiniveśa*

focus. See *dhāraṇā; dhyāna*

focused practice (*abhyāsa*), **29–32**, 35
inward (*saṁyama*), 40, 136, 241–244

Franklin, Benjamin, 179

friendliness, 221–222, 224, 251

G

Gandhi, Mohandas K., 143, 150, 171

Gibran, Kahlil, 165, 201

gift, 154–156, 162

gladness, 221, 222

Goethe, Johann Wolfgang von, 7

gratitude. See *santoṣa*

greed, 67, 144, 154, 166

guru, 72, 109

H

habitual patterns of behavior. See *saṁskāra-s*

Hazur, 217

heart-mind. See *citta; citta-prasādana; vṛtti-s; yoga as nirodha*

heat. See *tapas*

honesty. See *satya*

Hongzhi, 75, 109

humility. See *īśvara-praṇidhāna*

hypnotic trance, 236

I

identification, xiv, 33, 40, 76, 116, 130, 145, 161. See also *saṁyoga; asmitā*
  with the body, 27

identity, 11, 34, 161, 237

ignorance, 72, 73, 76, 108, 115, 144. See also *avidyā*
  removing the cover of, 22–23

illusion (*māyā*), 21

imagination. See *vikalpa*

inquiry/self-inquiry, xiv, xv, 125, 241

insecurity, 12, 113–116, 176

intention, xvii, 8–9, 52, 59, 60, 66, 67, 68, 107, 191, 196
  being careful about, 81–82
  of practicing *satya*, 150–151

inward focus. See *pratyāhāra; saṁyama*

Issa, 21

īśvara (source of knowledge), **43–47**, 162, 197, 201, 202, 204, 246, 250, 253

īśvara-praṇidhāna (humility and faith), 106, 116, 121, 125, 130, 172, 190, 196, 197, **201–205**, 246
  as part of *kriyā-yoga*, 185–186
  samādhi and, 237

J

Jobs, Steve, 9

Jung, Carl, 231

K

kaivalya (permanent oneness), 23, 50, 107, 110, 236, 242, 247, **249–252**

karma (action), xv, **49–55**, 146, 196, 204, 250, 253

Katha Upaniṣad, 218, 228

keen discernment. See *viveka*

kindness/being kind, xvii, xx, 3, 14, 18, 19, 49–50, 52, 76, 81, 95, 115, 124, 126, 137, 140, 141, 144–147, 155, 158, 163, 165, 176, 192–193, 205, 219, 223, 233, 250, 254

Kingsolver, Barbara, 95

kleśa-s (mental-emotional afflictions), 52, 76–77, 96, 99, **105–108,** 120, 125, 129, 136, 167, 186, 190, 196, 232, 236, 237, 245, 246, 247, 250
avidyā as field of, 109–112
asmitā, 113–117
rāga, 119–122
dveṣa, 123–127
abhiniveśa, 129–131

kliṣṭa-vṛtti-s (detrimental thoughts/emotions), 96, 106, 107, 231, 232

knowledge, source of. See *īśvara*

koans, xiv, 18, 237

Krishnamurti, Jiddu, 157

kriyā-yoga (practice in action), 40, 68, 76, 106, 107, 108, 115, 120, 121, 125, 136, 171, 173, **185–187,** 190, 202, 224, 246

Kṛṣṇa, 51, 218–219

L

Lao-tzu, 221

light. See *puruṣa; citta*

Loes, Harry Dixon, 249

Longfellow, Henry Wadsworth, 87

Luke, 49

M

Mandela, Nelson, 222

mantra, xiii, 45, 95, 195, 197, 198, 228, 243. See also *Om*

māyā (illusion), 21. See also *dṛśya*

McLachlan, Sarah, 123

memorization, xiii, 2

memory, 8, 11–13, 17, 39, 40, 49–52, 54, 76, 81, 92, 101, 106–107, 120, 124, 126, 152, 228, 238. See also *smṛti*

mental-emotional afflictions. See *kleśa-s*, 105–108

misperception. See *viparyaya*

mother, 22, 30, 65, 97, 211

Mother Nature. See *dṛśya*

N

nāḍī-s, xiii, 212

namaste, 18, 116, 203, 253

nature (inner), xix, xx, 15, 18, 27, 72, 97, 113, 116, 126, 135, 137, 140, 197, 209, 219, 232, 233, 243, 250

nature (natural world), 46, 57, 60, 254. See also *dṛśya; prakṛti*

nidrā (sleep), 75, **91–94**

nirodha, 3, 76, 77, 202, 203, 235. See also *yoga as nirodha*

niyama-s (personal self-care), xvii, 76, 149, **171–173**, 175, 179, 185, 186, 189, 195, 201, 202, 203
as second limb of yoga, 136, 171

nonaction, 51

nonattachment, 252. See *vairāgya*

nonhoarding. See *aparigraha*

nonstealing, 167, 253. See *asteya*

nonviolence, 3, 250, 253. See *ahiṁsā*

not this, not that, 18

Novalis, 71

O

obstacles that distract. See *antarāya-s*

Om, 45, 46, 103, 197
  as expression of *īśvara*, 45
  dissolving *antarāya-s* with, 102

one-pointedness. See *dhyāna*

open-mindedness, 85, 111

opposite, cultivating the (*pratipakṣa-bhāvana*), 165–168

oral transmission, 2

P

pañcāgni (five fires), 191

pariṇāma (transformation), **57–61**. See also change

past pleasure, clinging to. See *rāga*

past suffering, clinging to. See *dveṣa*

Patañjali, xiii, xiv, xv, xvi, xvii, xx, 1, 19, 40, 45, 71, 146, 185, 208, 236, 242, 253

peace, xvii, 40, 77, 136, 205, 221, 231, 243, 251

perception, xvi, xix, 8, 12–14, 22, 24, 40, 75, 76, 80–82, 92, 98, 109–111, 116, 167, 177, 195, 202, 212, 217, 218, 223, 235, 250. See also *pramāṇa; viparyaya; viveka*

personal self-care. See *niyama-s*

personality, 12, 13, 18, 28, 115, 116, 120, 171, 186. See also *asmitā*

philosophy, 3, 251

Po, Li, 235

positive influences, surrounding oneself with, 13, 50, 59, 223

prakṛti (nature), 18, 21, 22, 43, 59, 71, 73. See also *dṛśya*

pramāṇa (correct evaluation), **79–82,** 83, 85, 96, 104, 151, 197, 209
  clarity of *citta* and, 12

prāṇa (life force), xv, 102, 157, 207–208, 211, 214

prāṇāyāma (regulation of breath), xv, 19, 29, 100, 136, 175, 207–208, **211–214,** 241
  pratyāhāra as side effect of, 217–218
  as preparation for *dhāraṇā*, 229
  purification of the heart-mind (*citta-prasādana*) and, 223–224

pratipakṣa-bhāvana (cultivating the opposite), 165–168, 180, 223
  as antidote to violence, 146
  as other side of the story, 151, 165–166

pratiprasava (returning to the source), **245–248**
  eliminating *kleśa-s* with, 107, 125, 246
  ending *saṁskāra*-s with, 53–54

pratyāhāra (tuning out sensory input), 136, 208, 213, **217–220,** 235 as side effect of *prāṇāyāma* and *saṁyama*, 217–218, 241

purification of heart-mind field of consciousness. See *citta-prasādana*

puruṣa (pure inner light of awareness), **17–20,** 21, 22, 29, 33, 39, 40, 58, 71, 72, 73, 87, 89, 109, 175, 179, 202, 218. *See also* seer
citta and, 12, 221, 250
īśvara and, 43–44
sattvic citta versus, 250

R

rāga (clinging to past pleasure), 106, **119–122,** 123, 124, 196

readiness. See *atha*

receiving, 120, 153–156

regression, 99, 102

religion, xx, 18, 43, 45, 46, 197, 201, 251, 253

reputation, 84, 117, 129. See also *asmitā*

restraint, xv, 130, 223. See also *yama-s*

retribution, 50

returning to the source. See *pratiprasava*

Rumi, vii, 39, 65

S

samādhi (complete attention), 92, 102, 186, 190, 196, 202–203, 217, 231, 232, 233, **235–239**
as final limb of yoga, 40, 136, 235
as result of *saṁyama*, 242, 243

saṁskāra-s (imprint of actions/habitual patterns of behavior), 12, 31, 35, 44, **49–55,** 76, 84, 96, 120, 121, 124, 164, 167, 190, 196, 233, 245, 246, 247
diligent practice (*abhyāsa*) and, 34
nonattachment (*vairāgya*) and, 34

saṁyama (focusing inward),29, 40, 92, 102, 213, 223, 228, 236, **241–244**
dhāraṇā as part of, 227, 242
dhyāna as part of, 231, 242
samādhi as part of, 236, 242
pratyāhāra as side effect of, 217–218, 241
softening/opening of mind and, 18
as subset of eight limbs of yoga (*aṣṭāṅga*), 40, 136, 241

saṁyoga (false identification of seer with seen), 23, **71–74.** See also seer vs. seeable, 22–23

Sanskrit language, xiii, xiv, xviii, xix, 1, 2, 3, 4, 22, 45

santoṣa (contentment and gratitude), 172, **179–183,** 222

sattva/sattvic, 3–4, 92, 176, 177, 228, 236, 250

satya (truthfulness and sincerity), 140, 143, **149–152,** 153, 191

śauca (cleanliness), 172, **175–178**

science, 20, 21, 43, 45, 50, 53, 57, 84, 176, 204

seer, xvi, 18, 19, 21–23, 24, 92. See *puruṣa;* see also *dṛśya; saṁyoga*

self
  distorted sense of. See *asmitā*
  personal self-care. See *niyama-s*
  study by and of oneself. See *svādhyāya*

self-doubt. See doubt

sensory input, tuning out. See *pratyāhāra*

sensory objects, nonattachment to. See *vairāgya; pratyāhāra*

sensory organs, controlling. See *brahmacarya; pratyāhāra*

sensory perceptions. *See* perception; *pratyāhāra*

Serenity Prayer, 57, 58

Seuss, Dr., 25

sexual energy. See *brahmacarya*

Sheng Yen, 29

silencing the heart-mind. See *yoga as nirodha*

sincerity/being sincere, 30, 32, 110, 125, 181, 222, 224, 235. See also *satya*

Singh, Kirpal, 43, 119

sleep. See *nidrā*

smṛti (memory), 75, **95–98**

Śrī Guru Stotram, 79

Standing Bear, Chief Luther, 207

stealing, 167. See *asteya*

stress, 9, 19, 41, 176, 209, 212, 224, 232

students, xiv, xviii, 2–3, 8, 44, 88, 114, 181, 228

study by and of oneself. See *svādhyāya*

supernatural/supernormal powers, 242–243. See also *saṁyama*

svādhyāya (study by and of oneself), 35, 103, 106, 115, 121, 125, 130, 172, 185, 186, 190, **195–199,** 202, 246

T

Talmud, The, 83

tapas (practice causing positive change), 106, 115, 121, 125, 172, 176, 185, 186, **189–193,** 197, 202, 243
  part of *kriyā-yoga,* 185
  svādhyāya and, 196

Tecumseh, Chief, 129

Thoreau, Henry David, 161

transformation. See *pariṇāma*

truthfulness. See *satya*

U

ungroundedness, 99, 101–102

Upaniṣad-s, 197, 218, 228

V

vairāgya (nonattachment to sensory objects), 27, **33–37,** 41, 77, 101, 110, 141, 229
  abhyāsa and, 30–31, 35
  counteracting *rāga* and *dveṣa* with, 120–121

Veda-s, 1, 197

vikalpa (imagination), 75, **87–90**

violence, 67, 95, 143–147, 157, 251

viparyaya (misperception), 75, 80, **83–86,** 88, 96, 101, 151, 181

vital energy, conservation of. See *brahmacarya*

viveka (keen discernment), **25–28,** 30, 35, 58, 65, 69, 77, 80, 110, 136, 140, 155, 197, 223, 227, 250

vṛtti-s (activity in the heart-mind), 13, 22, 35, 40, **75–78,** 83, 92, 95, 99, 107, 112, 113, 115, 203, 224, 232, 245
  pramāṇa, 79–82
  viparyaya, 83–86
  vikalpa, 87–90
  nīḍrā, 91–94
  smiṛti, 95–98

W

Wesley, John, 175

White Buffalo Calf Woman, 11

Y

Yama (Hindu god of death), 130

yama-s (ethical practices), xvii, 76, **139–141,** 143, 149, 150, 153, 157, 161, 165, 166, 168, 171, 196, 221
  as first limb of yoga, 136

yoga as nirodha (silencing the heart-mind), 30, 35, **39–42**
  necessity of *abhyāsa* and *vairāgya* for, 30–31, 35

ABOUT THE AUTHOR

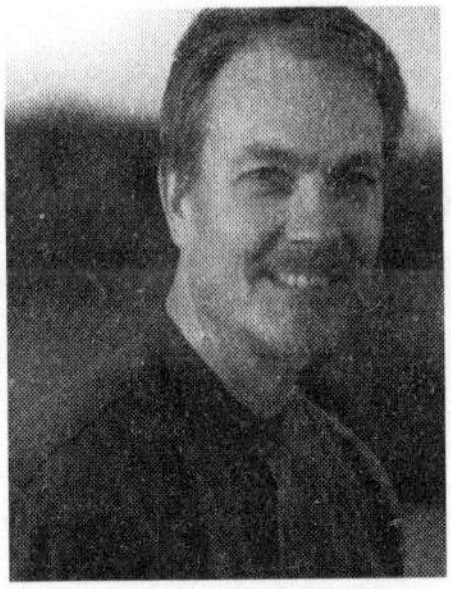

NICOLAI BACHMAN has been teaching Sanskrit, chanting, yoga philosophy, and Ayurveda since 1994. His studies with individual teachers in one-on-one or small-class settings form the core of his education, which combines informal, traditional study with the academic rigor of university classes. He has studied extensively at the American Sanskrit Institute, the Ayurvedic Institute, the American Institute of Vedic Studies, and the Vedic Chant Center. He holds an MA in Eastern philosophy from St. John's College, an MS in nutrition from the University of New Mexico, and is eRYT500 certified.

Nicolai's passion for Sanskrit, Ayurveda, and yoga philosophy infuses every class he teaches, and he has a knack for organizing complex scientific and philosophical concepts into a clear, understandable format. He travels nationally to share the deeper wisdom of yoga and to inspire students on their paths. Nicolai lives in Santa Fe, New Mexico, with his wife and children.

Among Nicolai's publications—all audio/visual learning tools—are *108 Sanskrit Flash Cards* (The Ayurvedic Press, 2009), *The Language of Jyotisha* (Sanskrit Sounds, 2010), *The Language of Yoga* (Sounds True, 2005), *The Language of*

Ayurveda (Sanskrit Sounds/Trafford, 2006), and *The Yoga Sutras: An Essential Guide to the Heart of Yoga Philosophy* (Sounds True, 2010).

For more information, visit sanskritsounds.com.

ABOUT SOUNDS TRUE

SOUNDS TRUE is a multimedia publisher whose mission is to inspire and support personal transformation and spiritual awakening. Founded in 1985 and located in Boulder, Colorado, we work with many of the leading spiritual teachers, thinkers, healers, and visionary artists of our time. We strive with every title to preserve the essential "living wisdom" of the author or artist. It is our goal to create products that not only provide information to a reader or listener, but that also embody the quality of a wisdom transmission.

For those seeking genuine transformation, Sounds True is your trusted partner. At SoundsTrue.com you will find a wealth of free resources to support your journey, including exclusive weekly audio interviews, free downloads, interactive learning tools, and other special savings on all our titles.

To listen to a podcast interview with author Nicolai Bachman and to hear the author chanting the Yoga Sūtras, please visit SoundsTrue.com/bonus/Nicolai_Bachman_path.

SOUNDS TRUE
BOULDER, COLORADO